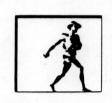

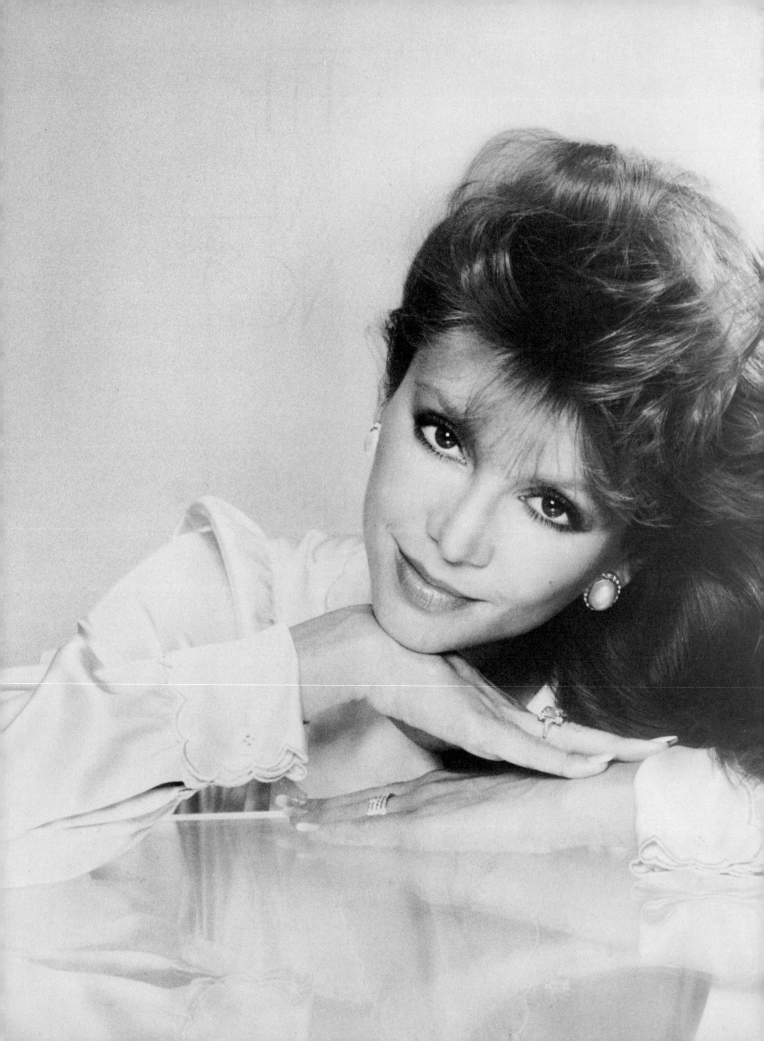

THE BEAUTY PRINCIPAL

Victoria Principal

Photographs by Harry Langdon

SIMON AND SCHUSTER   New York

Other books by Victoria Principal
The Body Principal

Illustrations by Glenn Tunstull

Copyright © 1984 by Pryce Hill Principal Productions, Inc.

Published by Simon and Schuster
A Division of Simon & Schuster, Inc.
Simon & Schuster Building
Rockefeller Center
1230 Avenue of the Americas
New York, New York 10020

SIMON AND SCHUSTER and colophon are registered trademarks of
Simon & Schuster, Inc.

Designed by Levavi & Levavi
Production directed by Richard L. Willett

Manufactured in the United States of America

10 9 8 7 6 5 4 3 2 1

Library of Congress Cataloging in Publication Data

Principal, Victoria.
   The beauty Principal.

   1. Beauty, Personal. 2. Principal, Victoria.
3. Television personalities—United States—Biography.
I. Title.
RA778.P9145   1984   646.7'042   84-13874
ISBN: 0-671-49643-3

ACKNOWLEDGMENTS

The following people made this book possible, and I want to thank them: Annie Gilbar, for sharing her friendship and her talent; Dan Green, the number one publisher in my life; Susan Victor, for her dedication; Jerry Edelstein, for whom there are not enough words of thanks; Leonard Katzman (for the time off!); Wally Bregman, my very good friend; Harry Langdon, for his ever beautiful work; José Eber and Marja Webster for the Beauty Principal "look"; Françoise Ilnseher, an artist and a friend; and Alan Nierob for a thousand reasons. Also for their invaluable contribution to this book, I am forever grateful to Aida Thibiant, Dr. Sandy Aronberg, Dr. Harry Aronowitz, Dr. Sonia Ancoli-Israel, Dr. Lee Hunter and Dr. Harry Glassman.

This book is dedicated to the one I love.

CONTENTS

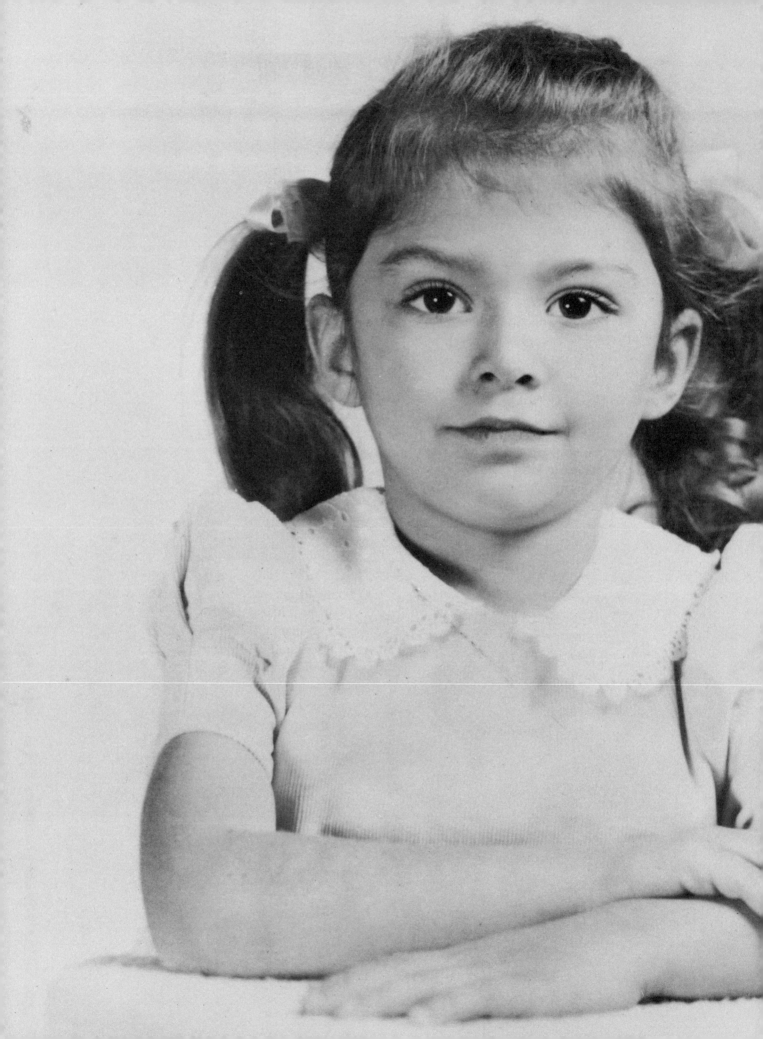

CHAPTER 1

BEAUTY IN MY LIFE

My mother is beautiful. She always has been.

When I was a little girl, I thought she was the most beautiful woman in the world: blond, blue eyed, with high cheekbones, long, narrow, chiseled features—a natural, classic beauty. She was my ideal. I wanted to look just like her.

But I didn't. In fact, it took me years to understand that beauty is not looking like someone else; that it is not having so-called ''perfect'' features; that it is not being a spectacular head turner. Today I know that beauty is being the best person I can be, and looking *my* best; that real beauty is energy and spirit and pride and humor. Being beautiful is feeling happy inside and being honest about myself. And then, with a little help from my friends—my moisturizer, my foundation, my mascara, my hair conditioner—and with a simple, enjoyable routine that takes care of ''me,'' I can make the most of what I have. And that makes me feel beautiful.

It wasn't always so.

When I was about four years old, I remember standing in the doorway of my mother's bedroom, mesmerized. I was watching her perform her daily ceremony of beauty care. She would bend toward the floor, stretching her body slowly and easily in some form of exercise routine. Then she would stand by the sink to wash her face,

My first photo session, at age four.

11

and then, sitting at her dressing table, she would choose from an array of creams and lotions, putting one all over her face, another on her hands, and yet another on her neck. It was a short, quiet, private ritual; I thought it was wonderful.

It all looked so important, but I'm not sure I made the connection then between my mother's beauty and the way she cared for herself. We would sit at her makeup table, playing with the colors, the brushes, the pencils and the creams, and I would pretend that even though my hair and skin were dark, my eyes were brown and almond shaped, my face was round—that I was going to look just like her when I grew up. I would be tall, blond and blue eyed, and I would be beautiful.

But as I grew older, I cared less about my looks. All I cared about was what I was going to do that day. My mom and dad learned early on that I wanted very little to do with dolls. I liked sports and I liked to play rough. I would be beautiful later.

Turning thirteen put a dent in my plans. I got the kind of braces you wear on the outside of your face. I was very thin, with this big metal thing on my face drawing attention to my looks in a very unflattering and painful way—and I hated it. I withdrew inside myself, and decided to wait it out. I figured that when the braces came off—then I would be pretty.

The braces did come off but I didn't look pretty at all. It was devastating, because I had really believed that what made me unattractive were the braces. When the doctor removed them, and I looked the same, I was shocked.

My mother kept telling me that I was pretty—but I knew she was saying it just to reassure me, to make me feel better. I wasn't buying any of it. I avoided looking in mirrors; I hated my hair; I had no interest in clothes. I just didn't want to deal with the ugly duckling in the mirror. How could I have been so cute at five and so unattractive now?

At fifteen, I decided to change the color of my hair. With my mother's approval, I tried a red rinse. At the same time, my mom and I began trying facials on each other which was great fun (although the one I made from talcum powder, eggs, and cold cream that stuck on Mom's face like glue was not a great success). I started to ask her questions about what she did with all those creams. I began reading the labels on her packages and looking in magazines that told me what "miracles" I could perform on my face.

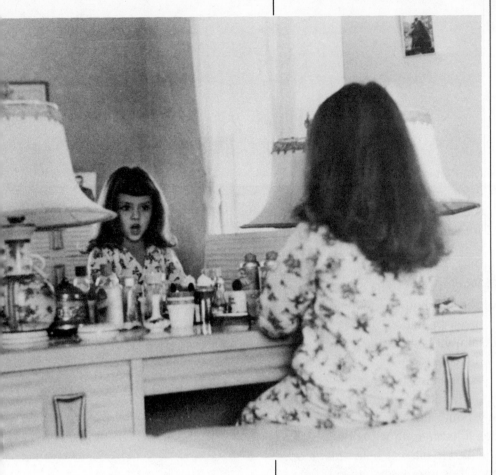

Caught, at age five, sitting at my mother's dressing table, made up and practicing for my future theatrical career.

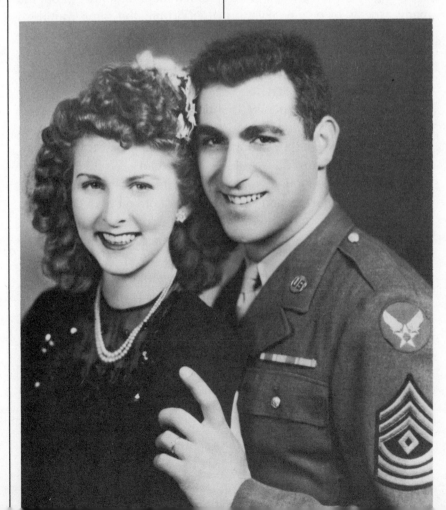

Mom and Dad

I experimented, I practiced, and through trial and error began to learn—even at that young age—about color, about skin and the importance of cleansing it (my mother, a fanatic about clean skin, once woke me up after she found I was sleeping with my makeup still intact). I also started styling my hair, developing a fascination with changing hairstyles. I changed my hair the way some people changed hats; it gave me the same kind of perk. Since I would get bored with a hairdo rather quickly, I became quite adept at creating different styles with one haircut. In between classes and after having done my homework, I would practice my new-found techniques on my girlfriends and on my mother.

I started to wear makeup in my late teens, and I wore a lot of it. I would put it on every day, religiously. Now back then we were talking Cleopatra—we wore heavy black liner, lashes on a strip glued to the eyelid, dark red lipstick filled in with yet another color and a heavy, almost masklike foundation. This was being *made up.* Soon I was making up for work as well because at seventeen I started modeling in commercials, where I learned more and more about the many aspects of beauty. Every day I followed the same routine: I would care for my skin, make up my face, redo my hair and try to be beautiful. I was told I was pretty. Men usually said I was exotic, thinking I would be flattered, but I didn't want to be exotic—I wanted to be "white bread" pretty.

I was grateful that people found me attractive, but I thought it was a fluke, and that I had better make the best of it because sooner or later they'd realize they had made a terrible mistake.

In my first year of college, I had a very bad car accident. I was lucky to be alive—and I knew it. I realized then that whatever looks I had—pretty or not—could easily be taken from me. I decided then and there to live each day to the fullest.

Doing commercials began to give me a taste for performing. So I surged forward to actively pursue an acting career. Also I promised myself—and I have kept that promise—that even if I altered the color and style of my hair, or plucked my eyebrows or wore stylized makeup, I would never forget who I really am, and I would never again try to be someone or something I'm not.

Today, because I am happy with both my personal and professional lives, my looks show it. I know that beauty starts inside, and with a little help on the outside, presents a total person. Beauty is seeing yourself as you really are—and liking the image that looks

Right: *On my first "real" date—that means the boy picked me up in a car. I was fifteen—the first time I was allowed to have a date. I am wearing some basic makeup, and my bouffant hair has been rinsed with a red coloring.*

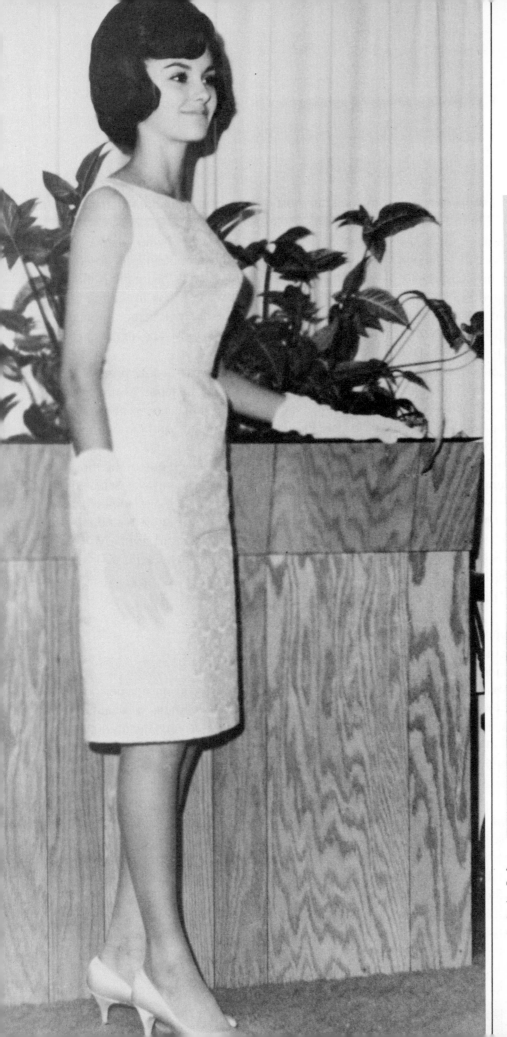

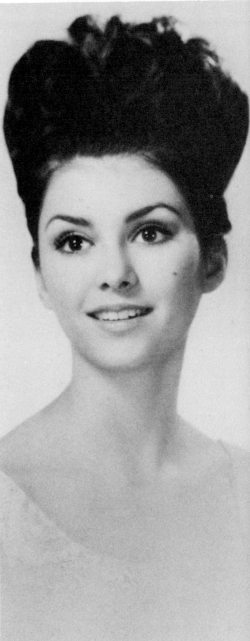

Above: *I am sixteen here—at the end of my sophomore year in high school. This was the "dressed up" hairdo. I have discovered arched brows and eye makeup.*

back at you. It is making the most of your own individual characteristics—and not copying someone else's.

In the business I am in, it is easy to lose sight of who you are, to start believing the stories and especially those photographs, forgetting the hours of work that go into making them as beautiful as they are. Nowadays I make a conscious effort when I look in the mirror to disassociate myself from the image—to really look at me. I notice the face, the lines, see what's new, what's old—and really take stock. I have learned to like what I see.

So I take care of it. I have developed a set of beauty principles for a lifetime of beauty, and have amassed a collection of tips and "tricks of the trade." I know there are certain things I need and want to do for the rest of my life to take care of myself. And I know how to do them.

But some habits die hard. In 1983 I was named one of the most beautiful women in America by *Harper's Bazaar,* and was selected to be on the cover of that issue. I was delighted—yet somewhat embarrassed. Still, after all these years, after the growth and the confidence and the healthy attitude acquired, I heard a little voice inside giggle and say, "See—you're still getting away with it. They still haven't found you out."

THE BEAUTY PRINCIPLES

The following lifetime beauty principles are based on my personal experience and form the foundation for becoming a beautiful woman. They explain that you have to work at your beauty now, whatever your age, and that you need to take the time to treat yourself to the essential luxuries of life.

1. Take Pride in Yourself

To be truly beautiful you have to take pride in yourself as a person. If you are outwardly pretty, but inside you are unhappy, or unfulfilled, or simply unrecognized, your aura of beauty will be somewhat askew. Imagine if someone gave you a gift wrapped in shiny, eye-popping paper, with glorious flowing ribbons and silk bows, but when you opened it, it was empty. You would be disappointed—

and the image of the beautiful gift would be destroyed. Even if the outer perfection is momentarily so dazzling as to be seemingly "perfect," remember, this perfection will eventually and inevitably fade, leaving a "less-than-perfect," inwardly empty shell.

The lesson, then, is to take pride in yourself as a person—let your confidence, warmth, poise, spirit, grace, humor—shine through. That is beauty.

2. The Pleasure of Your Face

Take pleasure in beholding your face. Let it be the mirror of your soul, your emotions, your feelings, your passions, your experiences. Don't be obsessed with lines and wrinkles—think of them as the expressions of your life. This doesn't mean you can't minimize them by learning how to take care of your skin, by applying makeup that enhances your best features, by wearing a hairstyle that is becoming —by making yourself as beautiful as you can be.

3. Your Best Is Beautiful

Beauty is making the best of what you are and what you have, and believing in your own beauty. A good friend once said that if you think you are beautiful, chances are others will too. Self-confidence is a large part of beauty.

Each of us has imperfections—eyes too narrow when you wanted doe eyes, skin sallow when you wished for a glow, hair thin and curly when you wanted it thick and straight. But what you think is a drawback may be what makes you *you*—it is the characteristic that distinguishes you from everyone else. This doesn't mean you can't, with knowledge and help, minimize some of those features you consider to be drawbacks and maximize those you love. But first you have to come to terms with your face and decide to make it as pretty as you can.

4. Be Yourself—Be the One You Love

Don't try to look like someone else. First of all, most of the people you see in magazines, in films or on television shows—those "perfect images"—are made up to look perfect for the camera, to be as beautiful as they can be for their roles. Believe me, their features are not perfect, either. It is an unhealthy waste of time to try to look like them because you are setting yourself up for failure—you can never look exactly like those women anyway, so you can never win.

Remember, those women without their makeup and hairstylists and wonderful camera people are just like you. Their beauty is calculated to please—it is not a pure natural phenomenon. Many of these women, when they look in the mirror, see lines and shadows and spots, just as you do. And yet, conversely, some of them are even more beautiful in person. Let me explain that one.

I have a very good friend who is also an actress. I can't tell you how many times people have come up to her and said, "You are so much prettier in person!" She used to wonder what the cameraman was doing wrong! But I realized that what people were really saying was that in life she has a spirit, a zest, a laugh, an expression that is hers alone—that is a part of her particular attraction. Her personal spirit makes her even more beautiful. It's a valuable lesson for everyone to learn and remember.

5. Being Beautiful Takes Work

Being beautiful takes work. Only in fairy tales are women born perfect and stay that way without any effort. But your beauty routine should be a pleasure. Taking care of your skin, putting on makeup, styling your hair, spending time on yourself—is not a narcissistic self-indulgence but an essential luxury to which you are certainly entitled.

My beauty routine is simple, effective and takes little time. But to make it work, you need the discipline of making such personal care a habit. To do that, you need to be *motivated,* for once you have the motivation to take proper care of yourself, you will want to make your beauty routine a daily part of your life.

6. Know Thyself

Take stock of how you present yourself to others, and make sure that what you *think* you project to people is what they see. Periodically I talk to my mirror and try to reassess some of my speech habits, my mannerisms, my quirks. Sometimes I find some newly acquired habit, and sometimes I find old ones I thought I had discarded. Part of being beautiful is having an image of beauty—that's what I referred to as having pride in yourself and a sense of self. But some-times our facial expressions and our physical habits give an unattractive impression.

We all need to see ourselves honestly, or at least as others see us. Part of this is noticing habits (are you blinking or squinting?), inflections and tone of voice (are you expressing excitement or are you screeching?), attitude (are you quietly attentive or patronizing?), and making a conscious effort to change or tone down the character-istics you dislike and enhancing those you consider attractive.

7. Find Your Own Style

After taking stock of the image you present to others, find your own style—one that reflects your personality and looks and fits your life. Understand the difference between fashion and style. Fashion is what designers decide we should be wearing, whether it is in clothes or makeup or hairdos. Style is your own special magic—an aura that is you. And it is something you can develop and nurture. Ask the professionals, look at magazines for clues to what would become you, what techniques and products will enhance your best features. In hair, in makeup and in clothes, you can find a style that reflects the way you feel about yourself, because style is an extension of your own individuality.

This does not mean that once you have found a style that is "you" you should be locked into that look. Have the confidence to be flexible, to try new fashions, but always remember not to be a victim of fashion—to let your own beauty shine through.

A woman of style is memorable and has an individuality that sets her apart from others. A beautiful woman has an attitude of self-confidence that radiates a style and charm all her own. She is beau-tiful because her skin is cared for, her makeup and hair are flattering, but she is also beautiful because she has humor, because she is honest, because she has a thoughtfulness and generosity of spirit that make her desirable and unforgettable.

8. Learn When to Break the Rules

Learn to break the rules—sometimes. Be flexible enough to be able to change. First learn the rules—how to care for your skin, how to style your hair, how to wear makeup that accentuates your best features and is appropriate for the occasion. Then learn when to use your judgment to bend the rules so that you are not *that* predictable. Sometimes flamboyance is terrific; sometimes being a head turner is wonderful; and sometimes being the center of attraction is wrong. Sometimes wearing no makeup is just fine, and at other times wearing an overdone face is just fine, too; but there are times when outlandish fashion is inappropriate.

You can learn how to set the tone for your moods and your needs. Flexibility is a wonderful asset as long as you know the basics.

Once you understand the beauty principles, you can then learn the practical, relatively simple and totally effective routine for a lifetime of beauty. In each chapter I explain the terms, the types, the problems, the solutions, the step-by-step methods of each beauty routine—and how you can adapt these to fit your needs. Each chapter includes tips, practical suggestions and "tricks of the trade" concerning skin, hair, makeup, bathing and other parts of the beauty routine I have formulated over the years.

I will also explain in each chapter how various special changes —such as weather, stress, menstruation, diet and travel—can affect your beauty life and how to handle such changes comfortably and effectively. There is a chapter on the many facets of sex and menstruation that can affect your life and therefore your beauty, one on plastic surgery, and one on the essential luxuries in your life (taking care of your teeth, your breasts, your nails, and so on).

There is a lot to learn about being beautiful—and the process is exciting and rewarding. Besides, being beautiful is fun. Just keep on reading and see.

In New York, while looking for work as an actress, I continued to model. Here I found a profession where beauty is everything. Little did I know how tough modeling would be, especially for someone who was not five feet seven inches, who was busty, who looked "exotic." But I was lucky enough to be able to work as a commercial model while I tried to get jobs as an actress. Here I am at eighteen on a modeling assignment in New York City.

Cattle calls became my daily nemesis—standing in a room full of other women, being judged not by how well we could act but on how we looked, was intimidating. I remember once being in a room full of young and beautiful women; one of them was Susan Blakely, who looked as tired and as distressed as I, with one difference —she looked stunning when she was tired and distressed! And she had legs longer than my whole body. That's what it was like then (and probably now)—a constant comparison of beauty among obviously attractive women.

After a while, this emphasis on my looks and the constant confrontations in cattle call after cattle call began to erode my self-confidence. The final straw was when I was up for the movie Goodbye, Columbus. *I was called back five times, and by the fifth time I was so nervous and insecure I was physically ill. I decided then that I couldn't go back again, so I quit—and went off to Europe.*

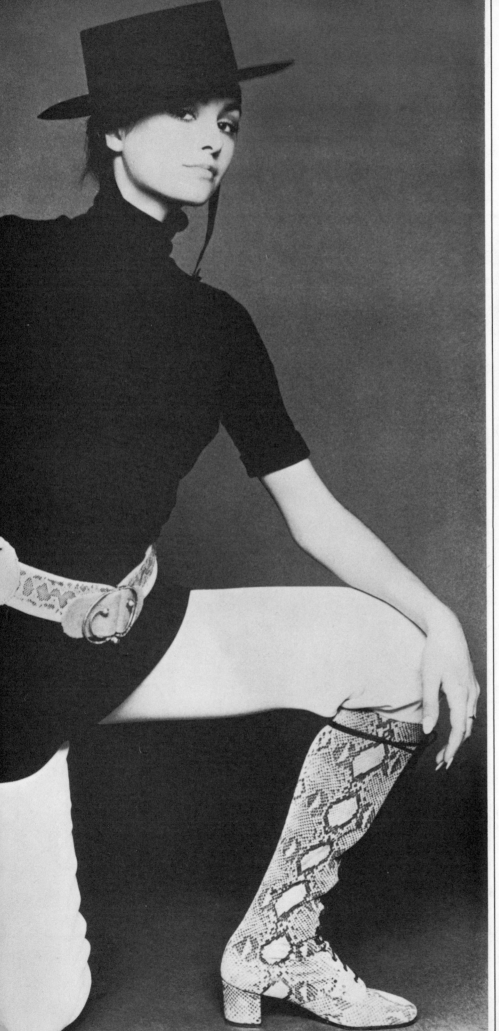

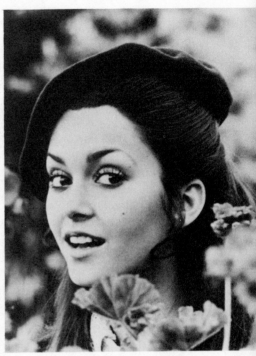

Here I am nineteen and living in Europe, studying acting with Jean Scott from the Royal Academy of Dramatic Arts and modeling to support myself. You can see by my sideways glance that I had learned that by facing in this direction in photographs I could make my "round" face seem somewhat slimmer.

This is a test shot for Vogue magazine, done in Europe in 1970. I did my own makeup for this shot but was helped by a professional makeup artist for the final touches. Although my face is still turned sideways to make it look thinner, I was learning about makeup techniques that would accomplish the same thing. I was also learning about skin care from European women.

The women I met in Europe were some of the most naturally beautiful women I have ever seen. They were not obsessed with how they looked—they just assumed that taking care of themselves, both inside and out, was as natural a routine as brushing their teeth. Their skin was clean and clear, their hair shiny, their makeup light and flattering. And, most of all, they were energetic, enthusiastic, and had pride in themselves and a joy for life. They seemed to know that taking care of themselves was something they deserved, something they needed to do.

Perhaps I was at a time in my life when I noticed these qualities, and perhaps European women really are so beautiful. Regardless, I was so taken that I began to learn their ideas and techniques and to digest all this new information about taking care of myself. I did it for me—and, of course, I knew that this would be good for my profession as well.

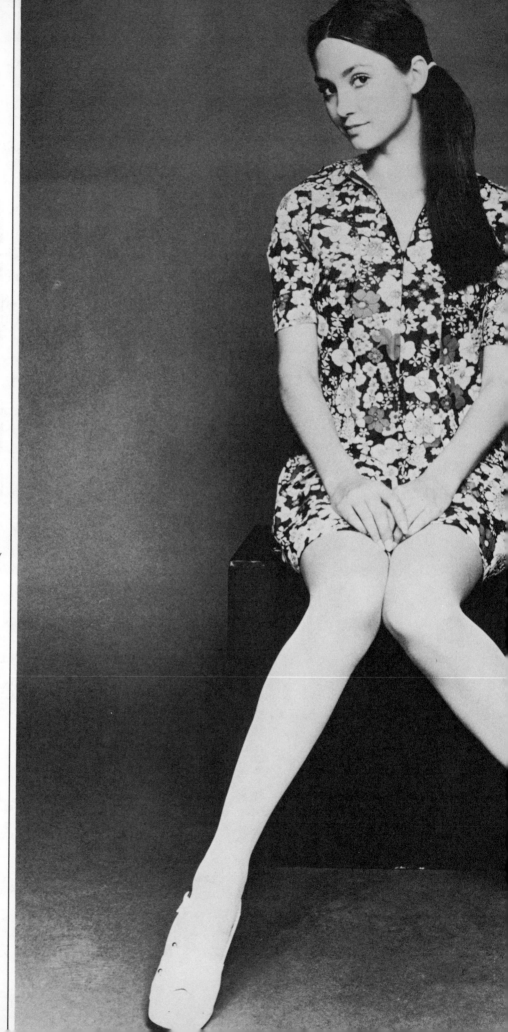

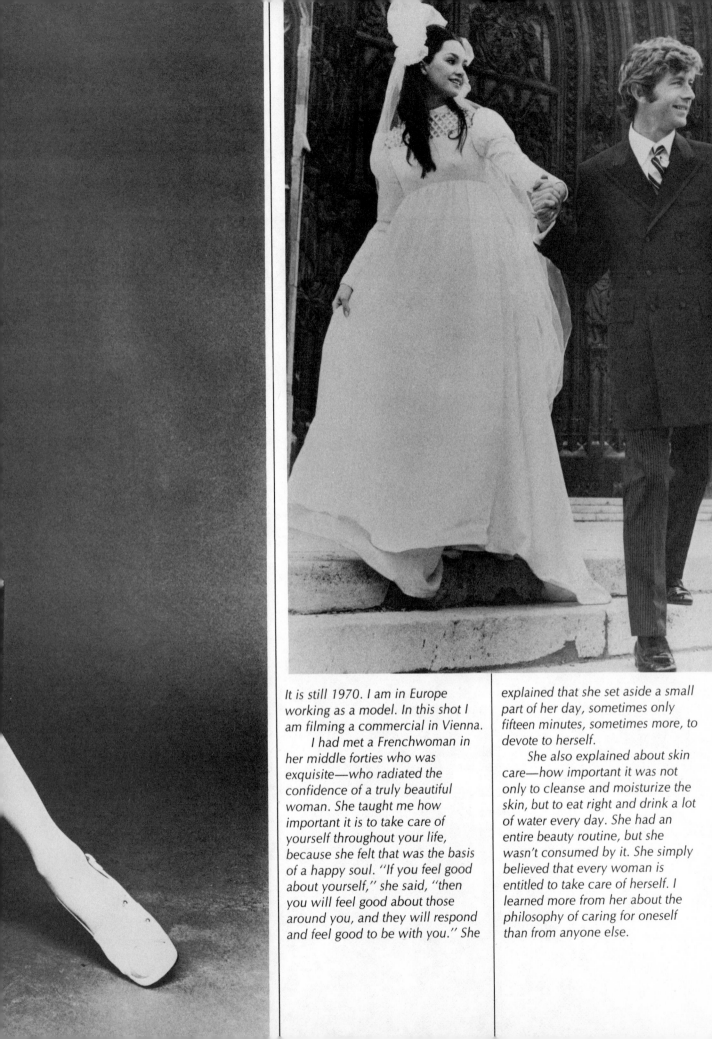

It is still 1970. I am in Europe working as a model. In this shot I am filming a commercial in Vienna.

I had met a Frenchwoman in her middle forties who was exquisite—who radiated the confidence of a truly beautiful woman. She taught me how important it is to take care of yourself throughout your life, because she felt that was the basis of a happy soul. "If you feel good about yourself," she said, "then you will feel good about those around you, and they will respond and feel good to be with you." She explained that she set aside a small part of her day, sometimes only fifteen minutes, sometimes more, to devote to herself.

She also explained about skin care—how important it was not only to cleanse and moisturize the skin, but to eat right and drink a lot of water every day. She had an entire beauty routine, but she wasn't consumed by it. She simply believed that every woman is entitled to take care of herself. I learned more from her about the philosophy of caring for oneself than from anyone else.

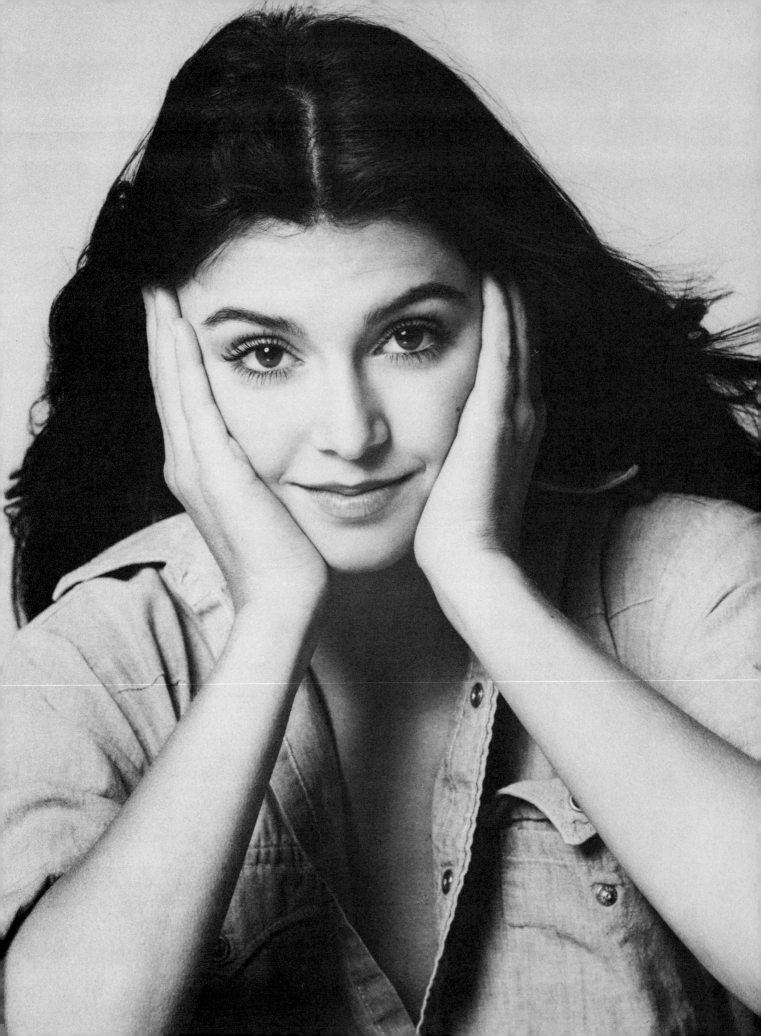

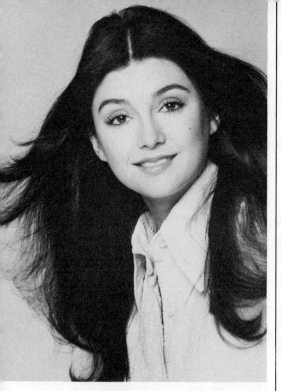

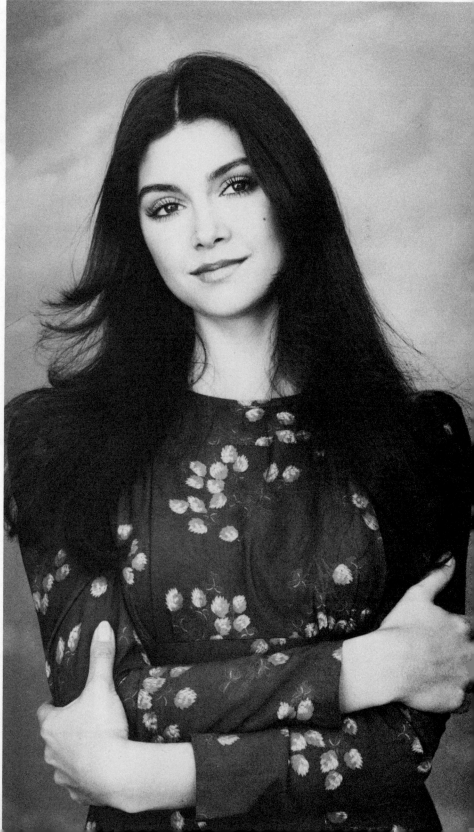

These photographs were taken in 1971 at the first session I had with Harry Langdon (actually, it was the first photographic session I had in Hollywood!). I didn't know what to expect, so I just brought myself, three sets of clothes changes, and no shoes. I did my own hair and makeup because I couldn't afford a makeup artist and a hair stylist. Besides, I really didn't know any better. I just figured it would be the natural me—unplucked eyebrows (unusual for those days), very little makeup and straight hair. I was extremely conscious of my round face, still laden with baby fat. Harry taught me to try various angles for my head, not just the three-quarter ones I had practiced. He taught me to use my hands to alter the shape of my face. But, as you can see, we also took many shots full front, round face and all.

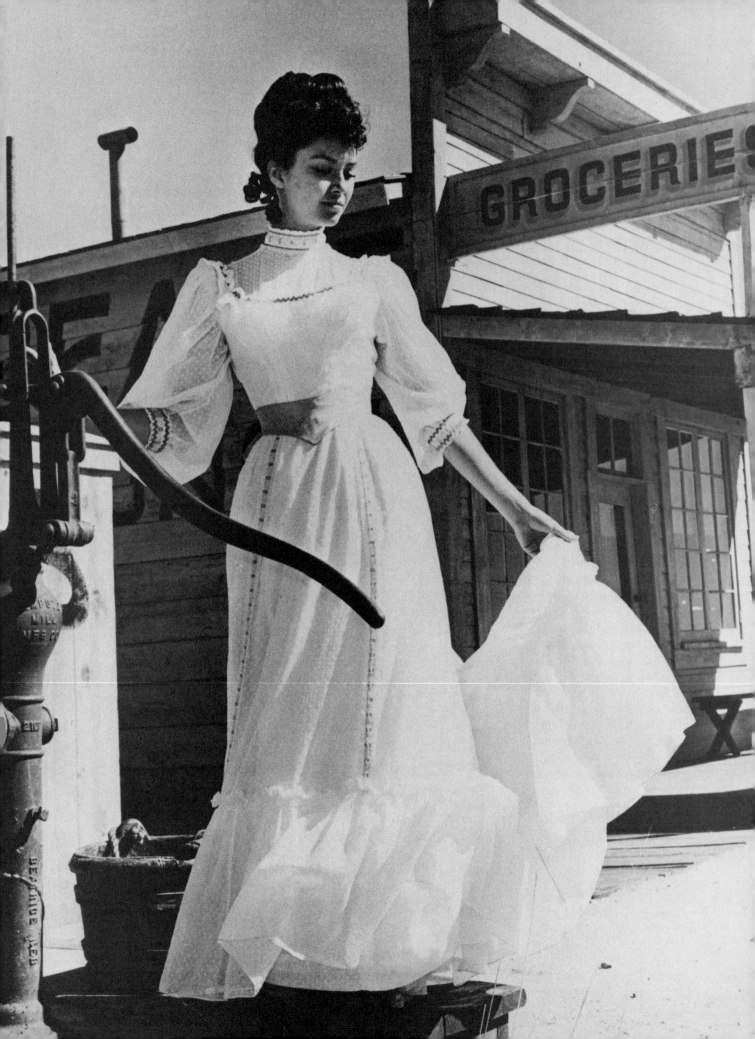

Left: *When I returned to the United States, I began to look for work as an actress in California. In late 1971, six months after I arrived, I was lucky enough to get my first movie role, a wonderful part of a Mexican girl in* The Life and Times of Judge Roy Bean, *directed by John Huston and starring Paul Newman, Ned Beatty, Stacy Keach and Tony Perkins. I became totally engrossed in being this unschooled Mexican girl—I let my eyebrows grow in and did virtually nothing with my hair. It was one of the few times in my life when I tried to get sun on my face to make me look darker for the part.*

We shot the film in Benson, Arizona—my God, it was hot! The new climate and my new daily work schedule made me grateful that I knew how to take care of my skin and hair, because this was the time they were really abused— every day, under the scorching sun, my hair was coated with petroleum jelly (to make it look dirty on film) and my face was laden with makeup. It may sound awful, but I loved it, because for the first time the focus was not on my looking attractive but on my work, and I didn't care how I looked—I just wanted to do good work.

Courtesy of First Artists Productions

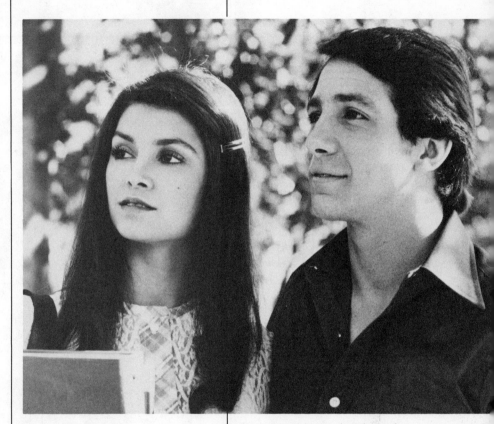

This is a publicity shot from the movie The Naked Ape, *with my costar, Johnny Crawford. I have straight, long hair, the natural makeup look and am still wishing my face was thinner. But now I am observing makeup artists and learning how to make my face look less round for films.*

Courtesy of Universal/Playboy

A couple of years passed, but my acting roles began to be sexier, not better, making me very unhappy. And, in my search to look like someone else, I became more and more confused. I wanted to be an actress, but as more emphasis was put on the way I looked, I began to lose sight of my work. And because I was always fighting my own image of what I thought true beauty was, I was befuddled, to say the least. I was still convinced, especially since producers seemed to want me only for my looks, that one day everyone would wake up and say, "Where have we been? This is a terrible mistake! And we thought she was pretty!"

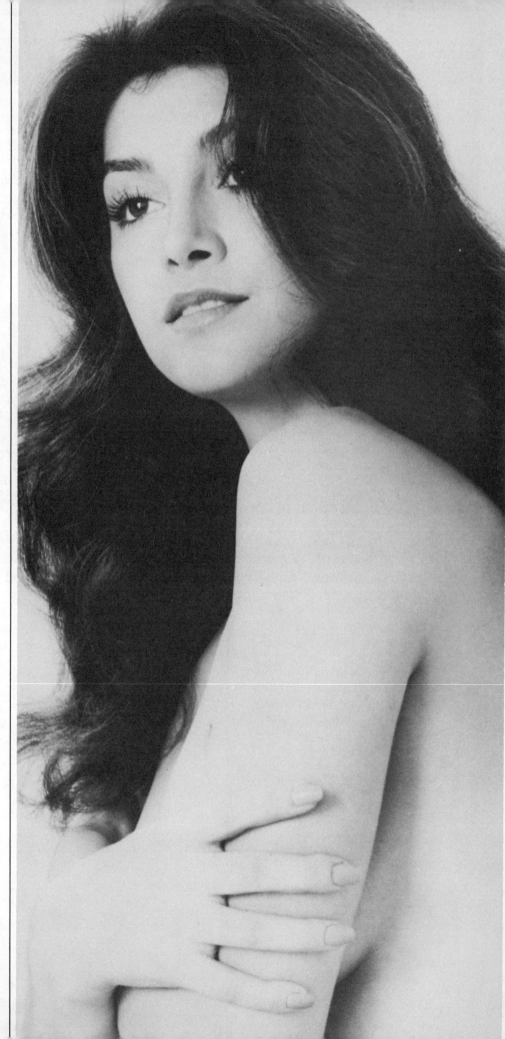

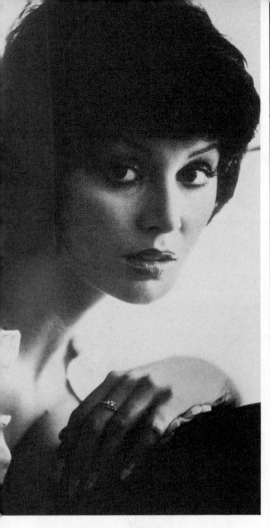

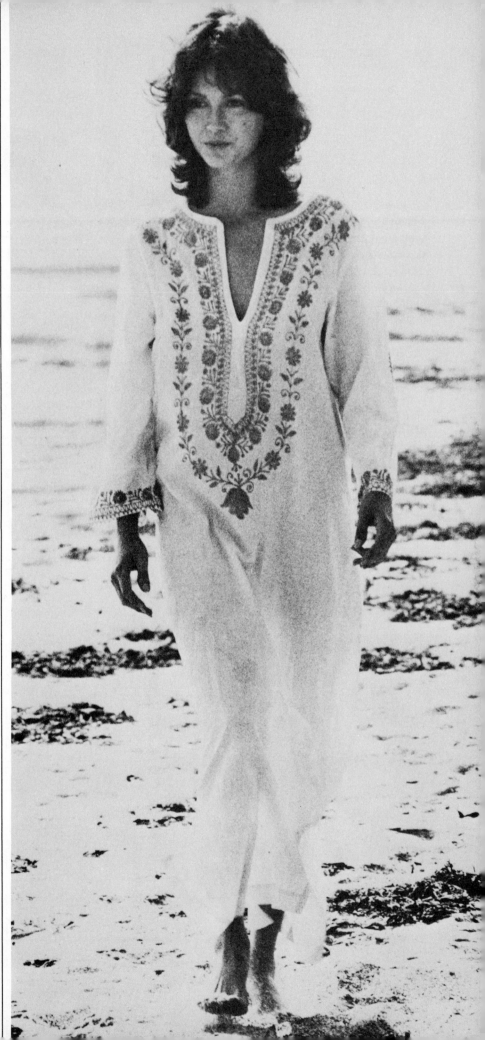

Above. *After* The Naked Ape *I wanted a change. I wasn't happy with what I was seeing. I liked myself as an actress, but I didn't like the way I looked and decided I needed something different. And that's what I got—for the first time since I was a teenager, I cut off my hair. Remember, it was waist length before I cut it, so this was a major change. I called it my Audrey Hepburn look.*

Right. *This was 1974—my beach period, the natural look. My hair grown out, unstyled, and I wore no makeup. I found a new kind of ease with myself, physically and emotionally. The only problem was I spent so much time alone I started to gain a lot of weight. This was a first for me!*

I decided to try it as a blonde, for a role in 1975 as a schoolteacher in Vigilante Force *with Kris Kristofferson and Jan-Michael Vincent. It was a disaster—not great for my hair or my looks. I had finally gone too far! My hair became brittle and started to fall out. Because my skin has a lot of yellow in it, the blond hair made me look slightly jaundiced. To compensate, I had to wear makeup with pink in it, and I had to wear it all the time. So I dyed my hair back to my real color.*

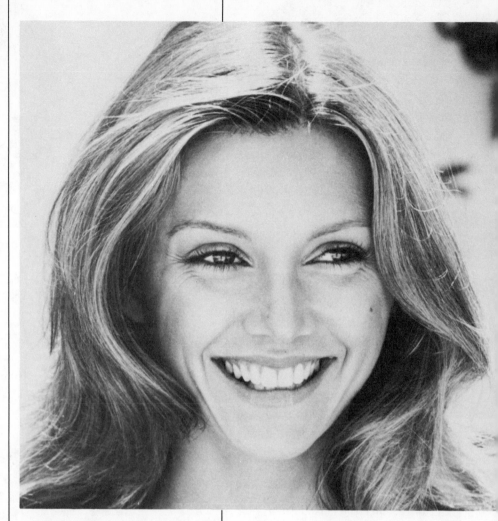

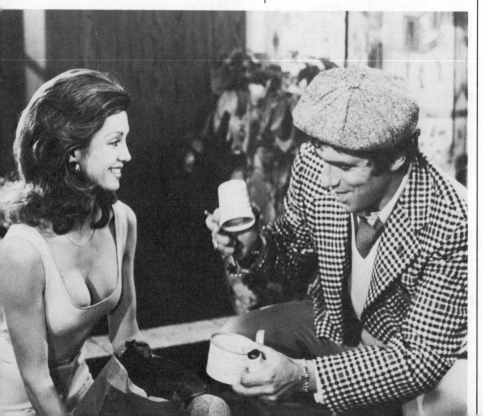

This is a shot from I Will, I Will . . . For Now, *a movie I made with Elliott Gould in 1975. It's another new look for me, one that evolved into a look that was mine. Something happened in my mid-twenties—my face finally lost its baby fat, found its bones. The roundness finally disappeared. I began to fit my face and realized that, notwithstanding makeup, this was me.*

Courtesy of Brut Productions

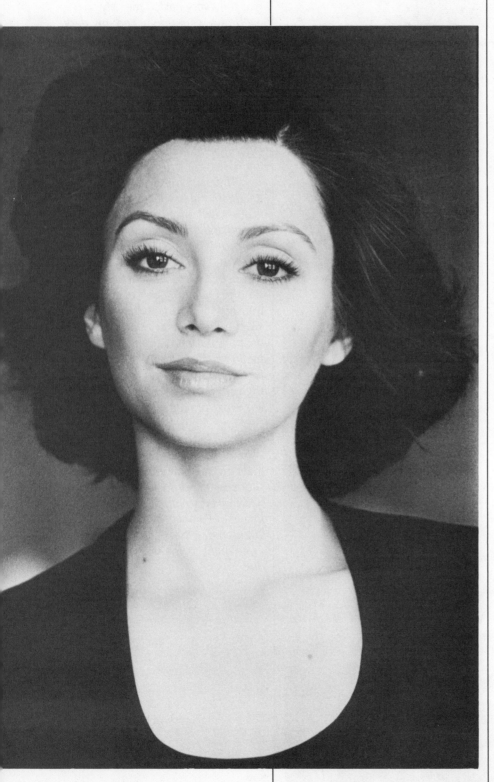

The focus on beauty, on how I looked, on sexy roles, finally took its toll. I couldn't handle being me —because I didn't know who me was. I didn't much like the ''public'' me, and the private me got confused with the public image. So I decided to quit acting and became an agent.

I loved my new profession and worked hard at my job. As for my looks—I cut my hair, figuring I would thus play down the glamorous old me. I thought it was appropriate because this Victoria Principal was a business woman and I wanted her to look that way —suitably efficient but not unfeminine. I wore very little makeup—only foundation, blush and mascara. I wanted everyone to forget the way I had looked and I think they did. Victoria Principal the actress disappeared.

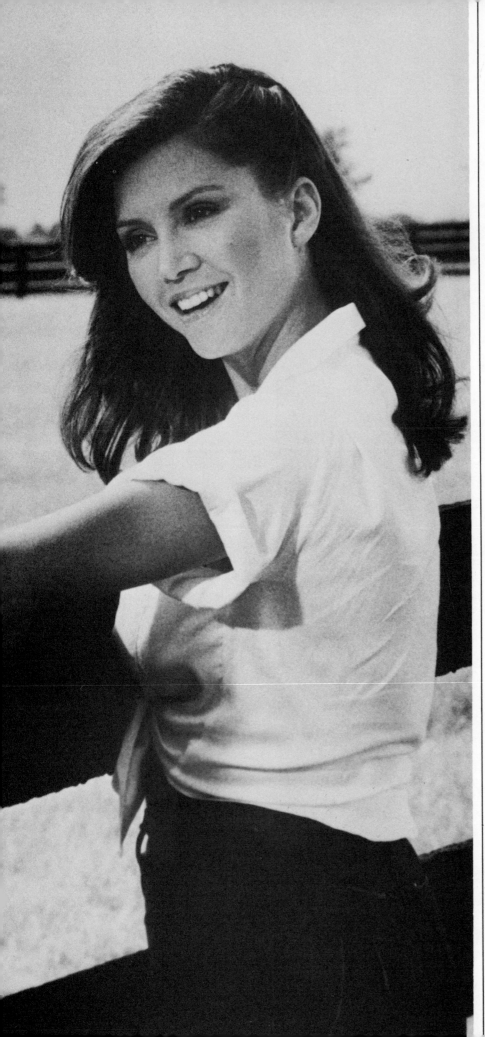

I resurfaced again in 1977, when, wanting to earn enough money to go to law school, I accepted a role in a television program produced by Aaron Spelling. Soon after I read the part of Pamela Barnes for "Dallas." I wanted it more than any part I had ever read. At the time I was the "very basic" me. My eyebrows were unplucked, my dark hair was one length and unstyled, and I had stopped wearing makeup.

It wasn't the best, most flattering look for me, but it was good for me emotionally, because I was returning to a career I had left as a "quasi" sex symbol, and I was determined to leave that identity in the past.

The day I met with Leonard Katzman, the producer of "Dallas," is one I will never forget. I was scared and enthralled. After endless hours of indecision, I simply went as I was. I wore almost no makeup, and my hair was straight and simple. I had on a pair of gabardine trousers and a forgettable turtleneck sweater. Later I was asked to test for the part, but I just couldn't do it—I had been away from the cameras for some time and was terribly frightened. So I asked if I could give a live performance, which I did. And I got the part of Pam.

I looked just like the "real" me —and I was the new Pam. As a matter of fact, on the first day of shooting, the producers decided I had looked so much like their image of Pamela Barnes on that audition day that I should wear the same outfit on the first show. And I did.

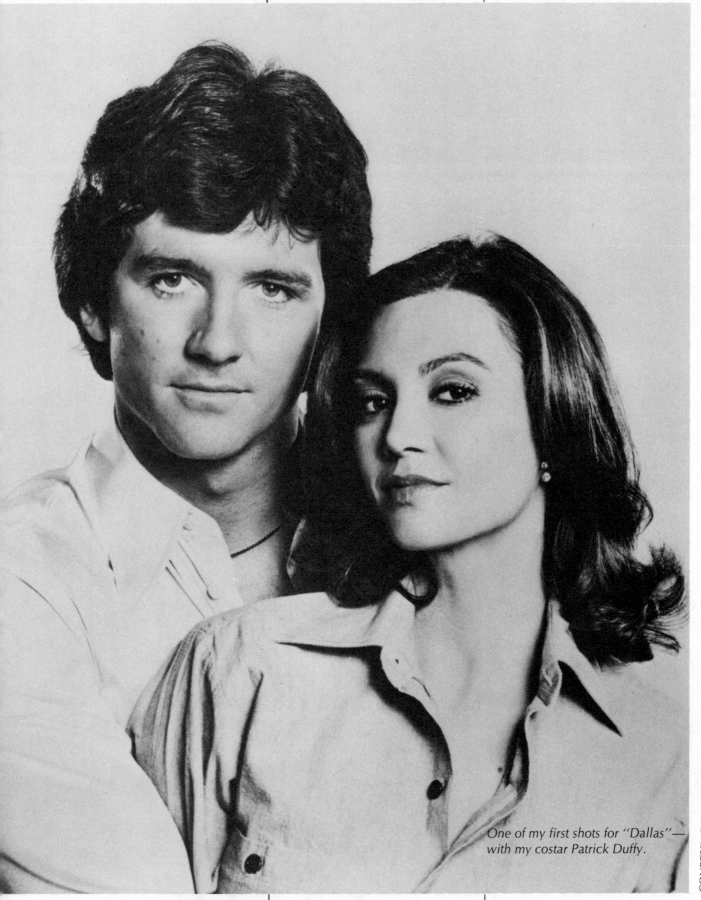

One of my first shots for "Dallas"—
with my costar Patrick Duffy.

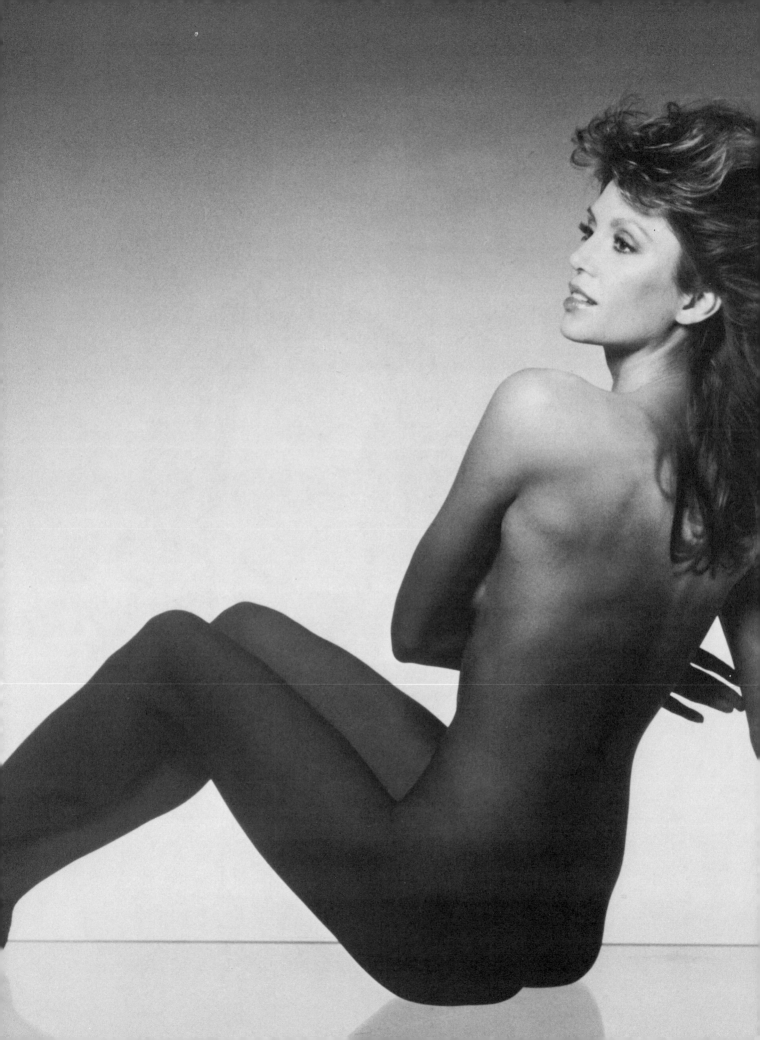

CHAPTER 2

A SKIN FOR ALL SEASONS

Taking care of your skin is the most important part of any beauty program. It is the foundation of a beauty routine—without it, the best makeup and hairstyle and exercise program will be for nought. The most beautiful dress in the world will not compensate for skin that has been ignored. But, on the other hand, wearing the simplest dress that accentuates clean, clear, radiating skin will make you feel and look your best.

Many times when people see a woman with beautiful skin, they wonder why she puts cream around her eyes, or why she goes to a skin care center, or why she routinely and religiously takes care of her skin. They don't realize that this care is precisely why her skin is so beautiful.

This is no accident—beautiful skin is not something to be taken for granted. You don't take care of it only when there is a problem, when the damage is obvious—you take care of it always. Even if you are born with great skin, believe me, it is going to change. That's a fact of life; so you have to take care of it now.

I have always believed that the condition of my skin, more than any other part of my beauty life, affects the way I feel about myself. And, conversely, the way I feel affects my skin.

Now there are times when skin is going to break out—when the weather changes, when our health has its ups and downs, during menstruation, when we are dieting, and particularly when we are under stress. Those are the times when the body's normal reaction process changes the texture and condition of the skin. These temporary conditions can be taken care of as the occasions arise. But daily care is essential to maintain your skin's health, elasticity, clearness and youth.

It is never too late to start a routine of skin care—but it's best to start young, in order to delay the aging process. My mother was right; she always stressed that if I took care of my skin early in life, it would be in much better condition to handle the inevitable lines, wrinkles and other problems of aging.

Skin care is a habit. It is easy to remember to do and as easy to do it, but it requires motivation to deliberately make skin care a daily part of your life.

Skin care is like insurance—do it now so it will be taken care of forever. Once you get into the habit of it you'll find it hard to break, harder still to disregard. And the change in your skin can be so immediate, and so rewarding, you'll wonder how you could have abused and/or neglected it before. If you take the time to improve the condition of your skin now, you'll also be improving the way you feel about yourself.

Just as your genes determine if you have blue or brown eyes, they also account for the kind of skin you have, the size of your pores and the number of your sweat glands. These genes are also responsible for how quickly or slowly your skin tans, if you are more susceptible to acne, and how quickly your skin responds to care.

But this does not mean there's nothing you can do to help your skin. The genetic makeup is intact, but taking care of your skin, regularly and carefully, inside your body and out, will result in healthier, more beautiful skin. And, perhaps more important, without such care, you can guarantee that your skin will be a mirror not of your soul or inner beauty but of the damaging, sometimes ravaging effects of the environment, weather changes and stress.

Our guide for the technical explanations of the wonder of skin is Aida Thibiant, of the Aida Thibiant Skin and Body Care Center in Beverly Hills, California.

THE PRINCIPLES OF SKIN CARE

What Is Skin?

Skin is the largest organ of the body. It is always in the process of renewing itself (watch how fast skin grows back and heals itself after an abrasion or a cut). Skin regulates your body temperature and helps the body get rid of wastes through perspiration. It protects the body from harmful outside chemicals and bacteria in the air, and from the damaging rays of the sun (although it needs some help here).

The skin has three layers, but we are concerned primarily with the basic two: the *epidermis* and the *dermis*. The epidermis is outermost and is made up of dead cells (they protect the live cells underneath), pores and pigmentation (color) cells. As those outer cells die, the skin manufactures new ones to take their place, usually every month (less often as you get older). The dermis, the lower and tougher layer, is made up of blood vessels, nerves, collagen, hair follicles and sweat glands.

When you are born you have "perfect skin," and it grows as you grow. When you are very young, your skin cells are healthy, and they get healthier (especially with care) until about the age of twenty-eight. It is then that the decline, or dehydration, of your skin cells begins. You cannot prevent this aging process. But with care, you can *delay* it by many years. That is why it is so important to start taking care of your skin at a very young age.

Skin care is preventive care in that it guarantees to lessen (not cancel) the damage that life inflicts on your skin. The fact is, there is no reason not to take care of your skin and every reason in the world to care for it now.

Types of Skin

I'm sure you have heard of the various types of skin you can have—dry, oily or "normal." It seems that wherever we turn, we are accosted by charts describing the characteristics of skin types and what we can do for them. Before embarking on any such analysis, you ought to know that many skin experts, including Aida Thibiant, have found through years of experience that 90 percent of the women they treat have "combination" skin, that is, skin that is somewhat dry

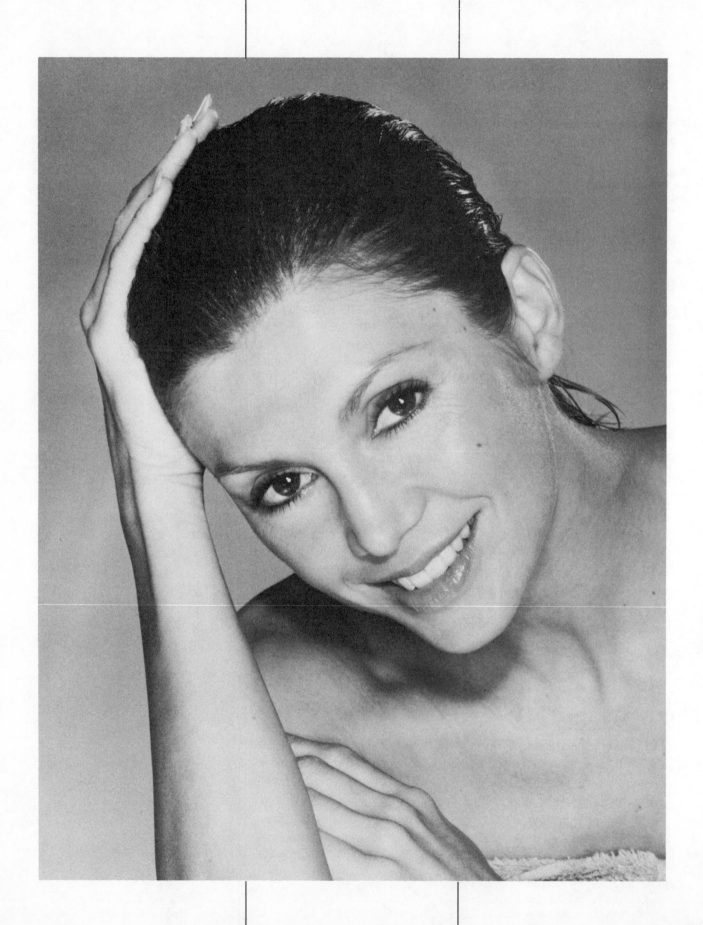

around the cheeks and the eyes and oily on the nose, chin and forehead—the "T" zone.

There are women who have basically *dry skin*—flaky, thin skin that wrinkles easily and can get dehydrated; or *oily skin*—shiny, greasy-looking, characterized by large pores, occasional blackheads and pimples. Women who have oily skin are always trying to dry it out—forgetting that oily skin stays young much longer than other types because it lubricates itself naturally.

But most women have a little bit of all of these and none of the extremes. As for so-called "normal" skin—well, the only people I know with normal skin are babies.

It is important to understand that all the creams and lotions and moisturizers and cleansers in the world will not change the type of skin you have. What they will do is change, through care, the condition and thus the appearance of your skin. But there is at least one thing you can do to beneficially alter the dry or oily characteristics of skin, and that is through your diet. (For tips on how to deal with your skin when dieting, see page 120).

Food and Your Skin

There is a direct relationship between what you put into your body and what shows up on your skin. What you eat feeds your skin. Thus it makes sense that by choosing your foods with your skin in mind, you can actually alter and help the condition of your skin. For example, everyone should drink a lot of water each day. It is not only good for your system, it helps keep dry and dehydrated skin moist.

If you have truly oily skin, I would not eat foods with a high oil content. These include all fried foods, creamy salad dressings and sauces, avocados, olives and the like. Healthy foods to concentrate on include vegetables, fruits and citrus juices.

If your skin is dehydrated, swallowing a tablespoon of mineral oil every day and eating nutritious foods high in oil (like avocados) will help. (But be wise—I don't eat mayonnaise because it is pure fat, but I do put it on my face to counteract the dryness of my skin.) Taking vitamin E may also help to lubricate your skin. Be sure to drink water, but stay away from caffeine, as it is a diuretic and will only further dehydrate your system.

For everyone, eating good, balanced meals helps develop a well-balanced skin because diet directly affects its texture and tone. Make a point to eat foods like bran which can help to flush toxins out of your body and thus clear your skin. Avoiding crash diets and harmful extremes of any kind will greatly help to keep your skin healthy and beautiful.

The Terms

What are these products that are so necessary to keep skin looking healthy and beautiful?

• *Cleanser:* Used to remove makeup, dirt, and some oil from the skin. It should not be used more than twice a day—overzealous cleansing is not good for the skin. The best cleansers are water based with no oil in them.

• *Astringent:* A clear liquid that lifts off that last layer of dirt from the skin, tightens the pores and neutralizes excess oil; to be used after cleansing, before applying the moisturizer. It usually contains alcohol which helps clean the skin and inhibits the growth of bacteria. It can also be used throughout the day to counteract any buildup of oil on the skin (see Chapter 3, Makeup, page 67). A *toner,* used for the same purpose, does not contain alcohol. You can use either.

• *Moisturizer:* Cream that adds water to the skin and seals it to protect evaporation; to be used after the astringent, on moist skin, and before applying foundation. Today almost all creams contain moisturizing ingredients.

• *Eye cream:* To be used on dry skin around the eyes; can also be used on your lips if they are dry. The cream is put on under foundation and at night.

• *Scrub:* Cream containing some abrasive (usually nuts, oatmeal or even sand) that cleans the skin and removes dead cells; can be used twice a week. Oil-free scrubs are better than those with oil.

• *Facial:* The process of cleansing, steaming, stimulating, nourishing and otherwise treating your skin; usually done by a professional in a salon.

• *Masque:* Made to stimulate and tone the skin, it also cleans and tightens the pores and removes the dead cells. You can do this at home once or twice a week. You can make your own masque or buy a commercial one.

• *Night cream:* A moisturizer specifically made for nighttime use; it is heavier than the daytime moisturizer and needs to be blotted off your skin before you go to sleep. You put the night cream on after cleansing your face and after the astringent.

Choosing Skin Care Products

Many creams and skin care lotions on the market are now made with nourishing elements, leaving out the harmful products that in the past were plentiful. But nevertheless it is important to familiarize yourself with the ingredients so that you know what to look for and what to avoid.

In choosing a cream, you *must* make it a habit to read the label —it tells the whole story. The ingredients are listed in the order of highest contents first, and least amount last. Thus, if you see a jar that lists collagen among the first three ingredients—grab it! If it has a fragrance first and collagen last, or if lanolin and mineral oil are first—put it back.

Things to look for at the top of the list on a label are any moisturizing ingredients, like water and aloe juice, collagen and elastin (natural proteins that keep the skin resilient), and sodium PCA (a natural moisturizer also found in the skin)—the so-called active ingredients. You don't want to use products with a high content of mineral oil or lanolin because these oils stay on top of the skin; they don't nourish it, they asphyxiate it, preventing your skin from absorbing moisture from the air. Another hint: Don't be put off by long names like propylparaben or methylparaben, preservatives that are in most creams to keep them from spoiling. If your creams don't have these additives, buy them in small jars and tubes, because their shelf life is short, and you don't want to have to throw away a half-full container.

SKIN CARE ROUTINES

Skin care is simple. The two main things to remember, the two musts about caring for your skin (especially if you are only willing to perform a two-step routine) are cleansing and moisturizing.

Cleansing

Cleansing removes the dirt, oil, makeup and dead cells that have accumulated on your skin during the day (but again, don't be over-anxious—removing all the oil that protects the skin from losing needed moisture will only dry it out). It is so easy to do—you don't need a formula, or special circumstances or a lot of time. You do it each and every night of your life. Period. No excuses. No "I'm so tired" or "My makeup has worn off anyway" or "I'll just do it tomorrow." To properly keep your skin clean, you have to promise to care for it every night.

Cleansing your body is something you do regularly each time you use soap in a shower or a bath. Cleansing your facial skin is at least as important, if not more so, and as easy. Cleansing your skin can also treat your skin, if done with the appropriate cleanser in the right manner.

Since most of us have so-called combination skin, the best cleanser to use is one that is water soluble and nondrying, a smooth cream that can be used with your hands, a face buff or a facial brush (you can buy a facial vibrator with attachments that are made for scrubbing and cleansing as well as increasing the circulation in your face). Such a cleanser will remove the dirt and dead cells without drying out the skin. If you prefer a cleansing soap, be sure it is not alkaline (which will dry you out).

For particularly dry skin, you can use a cleansing lotion or cleansing milk—but I wouldn't use soap; it might further dehydrate your skin. If you have very oily skin, you know that it can get dirty easily because dirt and makeup stick to it like glue. Be sure you use a cleansing milk that will remove the dirt but will not add any oil to your skin.

HOW TO CLEANSE YOUR SKIN

The nighttime routine when you remove your makeup is the beginning of any skin-cleansing program. For some people, their makeup remover *is* a cleanser, although they still use a separate one to remove eye makeup. For others, a cleanser can be used in addition to a makeup remover.

First, be sure to wash your hands. Then use a gentle, nondrying makeup remover. Spread it on your face and neck, and stroke it with your fingertips or a face buff. Be sure to use a circular motion and always move upward (gravity will pull your skin down soon enough). Then rinse off with warm water or a damp washcloth. (If you are going to take a shower, you can cleanse your face there either with a nonalkaline soap or with your cleanser.)

If you do this simple cleansing every night, your skin will be able to breathe while you sleep. In the morning, chances are all you will need to do is use an astringent on your face to remove any traces of overnight secretion from your oil glands, and then apply your moisturizer and your makeup.

There are a couple of handy and effective cleansing tools on the market now. One is a rough towel that is used to cleanse and rub the skin on your body. It is a terrific skin reviver and helps remove dead cells. The loofah, a hard, spongelike "tool," is also effective in ridding your skin of the top layer of dead cells. For the face, there is a gentle face buff which helps in cleansing the pores and also in taking off dead cells. You can also buy a brush specifically designed to be used for cleansing facial skin.

When using any of these "tools," be sure to rub gently, yet firmly, particularly on your face. You may need some practice to get this balance down, because it is important to stimulate your skin but not to stretch or damage it.

Moisturizing

The purpose of moisturizing is to return to the skin the moisture (not necessarily the oil) it loses naturally during the day and to protect it from the environment. Moisturizers do this quickly and effectively—with almost immediate results. If you have never used one, try it and after two days you are sure to see a remarkable difference. A moisturizer is a supplement to your skin (like putting a fertilizer in your garden), which needs moisture to grow.

Some people think that all you have to do with your skin is moisturize, moisturize and moisturize some more. That's just not true; all that cream could be clogging up your pores. First you need to wage a campaign against dryness and dehydration from the inside.

One way to do this is to drink eight glasses of water a day. This may sound difficult but is easier than you might think.

I drink a glass of water when I wake up in the morning and a glass before each meal. This gives me an easy four glasses a day. It also helps fill my stomach before I eat, so I eat a little less. I also drink water or diluted iced tea after each meal—to quench thirst and add another three glasses. Then, if I drink anything at all between meals—I've gotten my eight glasses of liquid. (For a more detailed discussion of diet and skin, see Chapter 3).

Moisturizing the skin on your body should be done after a shower or a bath (not in the shower or bathtub because you'll either slip or leave a slippery film for the next person). I use baby oil or a body cream made for this purpose, and rub it in all over. I then blot off the excess with a towel, and I'm done. Easy—all you have to do is do it.

CHOOSING A MOISTURIZER

Moisturizing your face takes a little more thought. First you have to choose a moisturizer that complements the kind of skin you have. Very oily skin may not need to be moisturized at all. If you have truly dehydrated skin, use a heavier moisturizer (you may also want to use a night cream for additional moisturizing while you sleep). For the rest of us, moisturizing is also a necessity, not a luxury.

There are many moisturizers on the market that include collagen. Try to use these—they can only help your skin.

HOW TO MOISTURIZE YOUR SKIN

After some practice you will get to know your skin well, and you will know when to moisturize differently at different times. When your skin is dry on your cheeks but is particularly oily in your "T" zone, you should moisturize only the dry areas and leave the "T" zone alone (or you can put some astringent on the "T" zone to get rid of the excess oil). If at other times your skin seems even in its condition and texture, use your light moisturizer all over your face.

The only rule is: *moisturize*. For most people, moisturizing in the evening and in the morning is the best idea. Do remember—after some education and practice, the best judge of how to treat your own skin is you.

Before applying your moisturizer, clean your hands and face and then use an astringent if that is part of your program. Now moisten your face and your neck with some tepid water (or with spray from an atomizer) because applying moisturizer on damp skin seals in the water. Now put a small amount of moisturizer on your fingertips and gently pat it at various spots on your face. Don't pull or stretch the skin—smooth on the moisturizer softly and carefully.

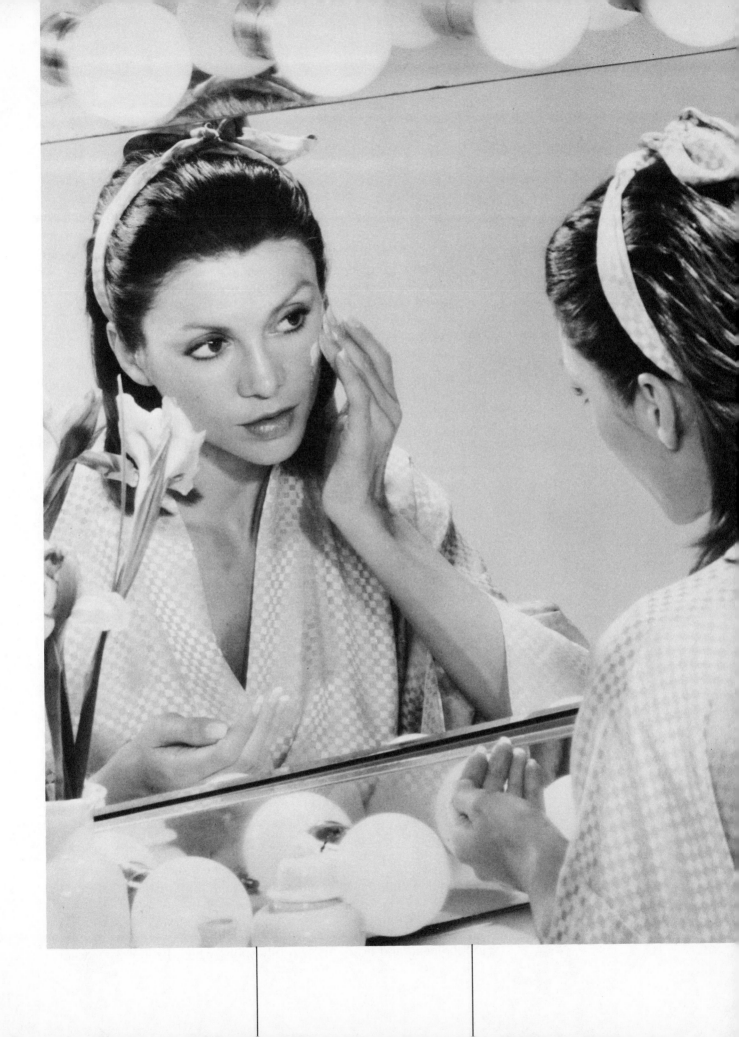

Now you are ready to put on your foundation or to go out and face the world as you are. Your skin is clean, moisturized and protected from the elements. An added note—if you don't wear any makeup, try to at least brush some translucent powder on your face after you have applied the moisturizer. This will give you added protection from the air.

My Skin Care Routine

Getting into the habit of a skin care routine is like anything else new —a bit intimidating and sounding a lot more complicated than it is. It's kind of like going someplace new—you don't know where to turn or what to do when. You have to try it out; it's a process of trial and error. But after a couple of days it will be easy. And after a week you'll be proud—not only because it will have become a pleasant habit, but particularly because you will see the results of your efforts. And then you will realize that skipping a day or skimping on the routine is only cheating yourself.

And it's so easy! The hardest part is getting motivated to start taking care of your skin. Once you are, the rest is a cinch.

IN THE MORNING

1. When I wake up in the morning I do some stretch exercises in bed to loosen my muscles and to get my circulation going. Thus by the time I make it to my bathroom, my skin is already somewhat stimulated.

2. I then take a shower (or, on rare occasions, only wash my face with a warm, wet washcloth). In the shower, I wash with soap and warm water, using a loofah to take off whatever dead skin is on my body, being careful to be as gentle on my body skin as I am on my facial skin. When I get out, I put baby oil all over my body (except on my neck because it will get into my hair). Then I pat it down with a towel.

3. Next I use a special moisture cream for my neck (because the skin on the neck is a different texture from that on the face). But using your facial moisturizer on your neck is fine, too.

4. Now I apply moisturizer all over my face except for my forehead and nose, my two oily spots, which I spray with water. I

also use a very light moisturizer on my nose. If I have only one moisturizer, I use it on my face and use an astringent on my nose to dry out the oil.

5. I use an eye cream to moisturize the area around my eyes. If you are not used to using an eye cream, just remember—it can't hurt; it can only help.

That's it. From shower to being ready for any makeup, the time passed is ten minutes.

AT NIGHT

1. I remove all my makeup with makeup remover, using a special one for the eyes, and put astringent on my face. Sometimes I do this at my sink, and at other times in the shower.

2. I put night cream all over my face, blotting it with a tissue so it won't be greasy.

3. I then put eye cream around my eyes, making sure not to pull or stretch the skin (I don't need any extra wrinkles!). Sometimes I put some on my lips—because it is an emollient it is wonderful to soften lips.

That's it. This took me about three minutes. Next time you want to go to bed without this routine, think about the extra three minutes and the results they will give, and I'll bet you decide it's worth the small effort.

Other Skin Care Procedures

FACIAL MASQUES
A facial masque is used once or twice a week to cleanse the skin more thoroughly than your daily routine does. It also refreshes the skin, tightens your pores and removes the top layer of dead cells more efficiently than you can with daily cleansing.

Applying a masque is simple. First you must make sure your face (and hands) are clean. Second, use your astringent to tone your skin. Now put eye cream around your eyes to protect that fragile skin. Then put some of the masque on your fingertips and gently smooth

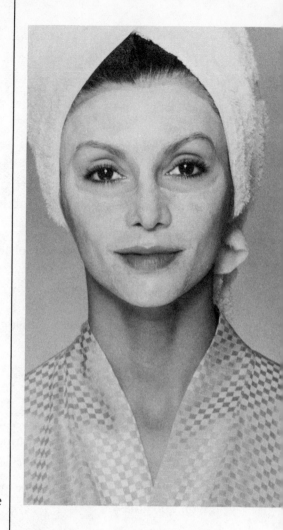

Facial masque

it over your face, stopping at the area around the eyes, and one-quarter inch from the hairline (you can also put some on your neck). As the masque is working, it will harden on your face. After about ten minutes, you will feel your skin tighten—that's the masque revitalizing your skin. It's a good idea not to entertain in a masque, and to tell whomever you are living with what you are doing—women with masques on do resemble ghouls.

Usually masques are left on the face for fifteen to thirty minutes (be sure to read the directions on the box). Try to unwind while your masque is on—in this way your facial muscles will also relax. I like to put on a masque while I take a bath; sometimes I do it while I lie in bed in the evening, learning my lines—when it is quiet and I can relax. When the time is up, I rinse my face with a warm, damp washcloth. I then apply my astringent and moisturizer—and go to bed.

Commercial masques are available at drugstores, skin care centers and the cosmetic sections of department stores. If you prefer, you can make your own masques at home. Two of my favorites are:

1. Take equal parts (one tablespoon will do) of yogurt and honey; add one egg yolk, and mix gently. Let it stand at room tem-

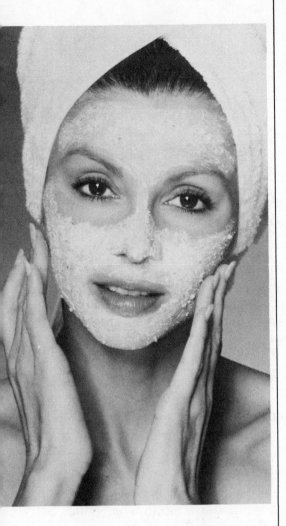

Facial scrub

perature so it is not cold. Now apply the mixture to your face as per the instructions above. Let it stay on your face for twenty minutes.

2. Another favorite is made from avocados. Simply blend an avocado in a blender or food processor, adding a few drops of lemon (this acts as an astringent which will tighten your pores). Then put it on your face, leaving it on for twenty minutes. Be sure to tone and moisturize when you are done.

Now what could be easier?

FACIAL SCRUBS
The purpose of a scrub is to clean and to remove the dead cells on your skin. This is done by putting the scrub on your clean fingertips and gently massaging your face. When you have done this for a minute or so, rinse with warm water. I use my scrub in the shower— my pores are open from the steam, so I know I am getting my skin as clean as possible.

There are commercial scrubs available, many with chopped nuts in them. I also make my own—using a one-quarter cup of oatmeal mixed with a little water or yogurt. When I am done, I use my astringent and moisturizer, just as I do after a masque.

The nice thing about scrubs is that they can be used as often as you like on any type of skin (unless you have extremely sensitive skin). Try giving your hands the scrub treatment, finishing off with a hand cream.

FACIALS

Facials—the process by which one cleans and conditions the skin—are most often done by professionals. I think it's a great idea to see a professional skin care technician or specialist at least once a year, and getting a facial is the perfect opportunity. These professionals will help you to understand your skin and teach you how to treat it at home. A good skin care technician will not make you dependent on her—she will help to make you the best expert on your skin.

Having a facial is a private, totally relaxing procedure where a licensed expert will spend more than one hour going over your skin with the utmost care. The process includes special and deep cleansing of the pores (including steaming your face); removal of blackheads; brushing with an electric brush and a scrub to remove the dead cells; massaging the skin to increase circulation; applying a masque to close the pores and tighten the skin; using a warm masque to moisturize dehydrated areas; and a final oil or moisturizer as the finishing touch. When it's over, you will feel rejuvenated, as if someone has given you a new skin.

Such facials are excellent for the skin but can be considered a luxury. Although I do have professional facials occasionally, I have developed a method to do them for myself at home.

THE HOME FACIAL

1. I begin by steaming my face with a portable steam machine. You can also take a warm-to-hot, soaking-wet washcloth and apply it to your face to open the pores of your skin. If you have an enclosed shower, you can get a similar effect by letting the steam build up.

2. Now use your facial scrub, as described earlier, cleaning your entire face (except for the eyes). Be sure to include your "lip line"—blackheads often hide there.

3. While your skin is moist and your pores are open, you can try to remove a blackhead that seems to be near the surface of your

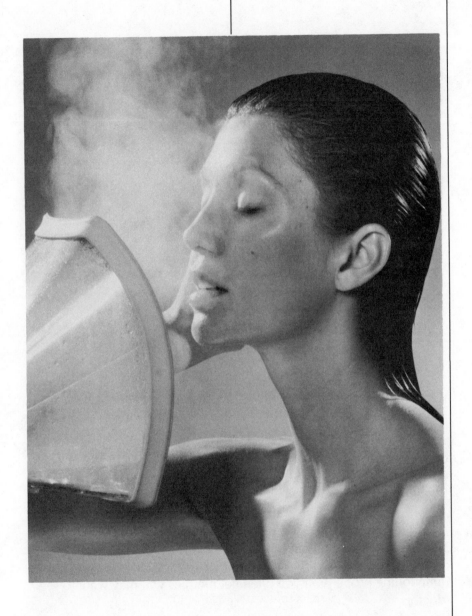

skin (leave the others alone!). Take your fingertips and gently squeeze the blackhead—first from two directions, then from the other two directions. Don't squeeze hard or you'll end up with broken capillaries. If you can't get the blackhead out, leave it alone.

4. Now use your cleanser.

5. Use either a masque or put warm oil on your face, for added moisturizing.

6. Splash on some cold water to close your facial pores.

7. End with a light moisturizer on your face, and your eye cream around your eyes.

That's it. Your home facial should take about thirty minutes. Set aside this private time to take special care of your skin. Do it when you are home alone, when you aren't in a hurry. Turn on some soothing music; don't answer the phone. Enjoy your moments alone —and heal your skin at the same time.

If you have the time and inclination to give yourself a facial once a week—that's great. For others, once a month is much better than a poke in the eye, as they say.

SPECIAL SKIN PROBLEMS

Pimples

I would guess that like me, many of you have a common problem— a pimple that pops up at the most inappropriate and inopportune moment (actually, any time a pimple pops up is inappropriate). Be that as it may, pimples appear. And they have to be handled.

Step one is to know that a blackhead pimple, the most common of all, is oil that got clogged in the pore and, when it oxidized with the air, turned black. If this blackhead gets infected, it can turn into a pimple. But a pimple can also be a symptom of an internal problem: You ate too much greasy food and your body couldn't digest all that oil, so it secreted it through the skin; or your liver may not be functioning properly. If you often get pimples you may want to see a doctor.

Step two is to decide that the pimple is not a tragedy, that it is probably more noticeable to you than it is to those around you.

Step three is to take charge. Try to find out why you got the pimple, because some causes are treatable. Here are some examples:

• Perhaps you have been under some sort of stress that can be channeled elsewhere (how about exercise?); many women under stress produce more oil which can result in a breakout.

• Perhaps you are about to menstruate; when a woman menstruates, there is a hormonal change in her system which often shows up on her face. It is common—and it is easy to handle because you know it will happen each month, and you know the cause. Aida Thibiant recommends cleaning your face more often and with more regularity so that the unclogged pores will allow the flow of oil to come out more freely, leaving your pores extra clean.

• Changes in diet can also cause a skin breakout.

Step four is to treat the pimple. The rule is—don't pick at it. It may get larger, it may bleed, it may get infected, and it *will* get uglier. I try a couple of things. Sometimes I take a cotton swab and dip it in alcohol or in my astringent. I then apply it to my pimple, put some medicated coverup on it, and go on with my life, knowing that I look as good as I can and that I am healing my skin in the process.

Sometimes I mix a tablespoon of cornstarch with a touch of alcohol (and rosewater, if you have it), and put a drop on the pimple. It will dry, so leave it there for thirty minutes; then wash it off (if you prefer, you can sleep with the mixture on the pimple—it will reduce the redness and you can remove it in the morning). I also buy a drying stick (you can find one in any drugstore) and keep it with my skin care products. That way I always have it handy when I need it.

If I am ready to go to bed and I want the pimple to come to a head, I take a warm washcloth and press the area until the blackhead is extracted. Then I put some alcohol and some medicine on it and go to sleep.

You might try to remember that getting a pimple is nature's way of releasing oil from your body, or telling you that something is haywire in your system. Pay attention to the signs, control whatever you can, and calmly deal with the problem. And go out and face the world—don't powder the you-know-what into oblivion; don't put extra foundation on it to call everyone's attention to it. Just take care of it—and remember that these pimples are temporary—chances are they'll be gone by morning.

Skin Spots

There are skin blemishes, broken capillaries and discolorations that can be treated; they can also be prevented if you know the cause.

Yellow discoloration of the skin (that is not jaundice caused by a liver problem) can be caused by smoking. Nicotine gives your skin a yellowish cast—which should be an additional incentive not to smoke.

Broken capillaries can be caused by drinking too much alcohol. Ever notice how someone who drinks too much liquor has red splotches on the cheeks and the nose? These are broken capillaries or blood vessels, and they have been linked to alcohol consumption. Do yourself a favor—stick to wine or an occasional Scotch.

Other causes of broken capillaries are eating too much spicy food and living in areas of extreme temperatures. In the latter, where people go from hot heat at home to cold outdoor temperatures, skin with broken capillaries is common. The only thing to do is to protect your skin—clean and moisturize faithfully; try not to go outside with damp skin; and cover your face in extremely cold temperatures.

Skin spots have several causes. One is taking birth control pills. Another is sun, which causes "sun spots" on your skin to darken and/or get larger. These spots can be bleached and removed by a dermatologist, but you can avoid them by staying out of the sun, especially without protection and when you are taking any medication, particularly an antibiotic or a sulfa drug. Ask your doctor if the medication you are taking can make your skin sensitive to the sun.

Another reason for sun spots may surprise you—perfume. Putting perfume on your face or neck before going out into the sun may cause a "photosensitive" reaction which results in spots on your skin.

Other skin blemishes can be caused by allergies. I have a friend in her thirties who, three years ago, suddenly developed acne. She went to numerous doctors and no one could discover the cause of the problem. But, smart lady that she is—she discovered it on her own. A couple of months ago she got rid of her pillows and bought new ones, just as a redecorating step. The day she threw out the old pillows, her skin cleared up.

Thus, if you suddenly develop a skin reaction—small, hard pimples that seem to sprout up overnight—see a doctor, but also try to figure out if there is anything you are doing that is different from your routine. Are you wearing a new fabric, using a new detergent, spending more time around animals, using a new cosmetic—all of these can cause reactions on your skin. And what's more aggravating and puzzling—you can suddenly develop an allergy to something you have been using for a very long time, whether it's a skin care product or a pillow. So be aware that allergies can show up on your skin. Try to localize the source—and then treat your skin.

Wrinkles

Everybody has some wrinkles, and once you have them, you have them. You won't be able to give them away, no matter how hard you try. That is why preventive skin care is so essential—you can delay and prevent premature wrinkle lines on your face if you care for your skin all your life, starting at a young age.

Premature wrinkles are caused by stretching the skin, by exposure to ultraviolet rays of the sun, by stress in your life, by lack of sleep, by dry skin and by heredity.

What you can do for wrinkles—other than try to remove them with plastic surgery, which is only successful with some kinds of facial lines—is to keep them moisturized, because the moisture is absorbed by the skin and fills out the lines. This simply means keeping your skin moisturized as in the skin routine—it does not mean you should smear globs of oil on your skin, hoping to fill in or erase years of abuse and neglect. Many women figure they'll put oil on their faces, go to bed and their wrinkles will diminish, if not disappear. What actually happens is that they wake up with a puffy face, sometimes a slightly swollen one—and that is why the lines seem to go away. And, like all short-term remedies, the swelling will go down, and the lines will return.

The things *to do* include the following:

1. You can wear a sun block to protect your face from the sun so the wrinkles and lines won't get worse.

2. You can avoid crash diets which stretch out the skin.

3. You can try not to sleep on your face, which also stretches the skin.

4. You can use creams with collagen, which nourish your skin and fill it in.

5. You can use light, moisturized foundation—heavy coverup will only accentuate the wrinkles.

6. You can embark on a simple skin care routine that will keep your skin in as good condition as possible.

A word about facial expressions. It is true that facial mannerisms can cause facial lines. My feeling is—worry only if these expressions are truly exaggerated. If you pull or pucker your lips all the time, if you wrinkle your forehead regularly, if you wiggle your nose every day, if you squint those eyes—these are things you can minimize and control.

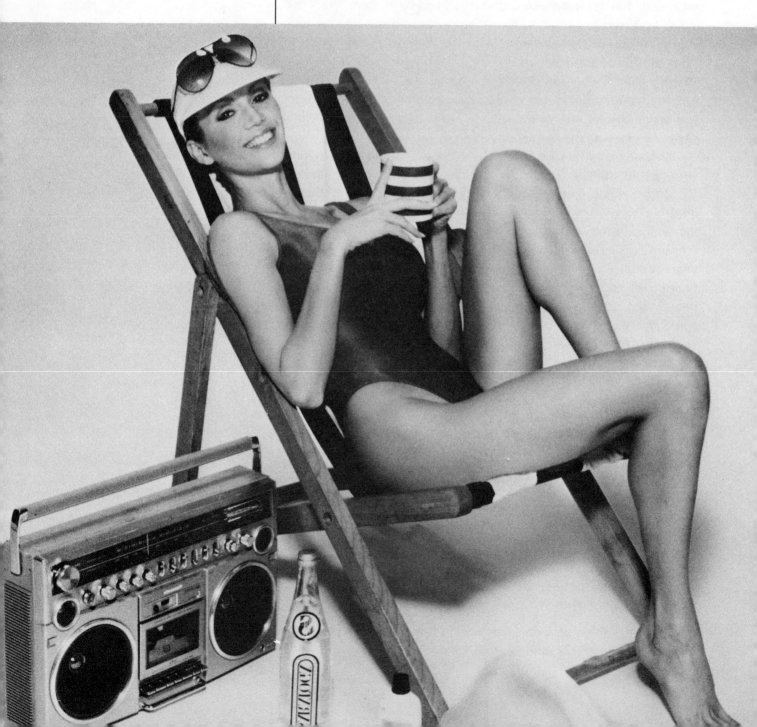

But don't stop laughing, or crying, or otherwise letting life show on your face. Our faces are the sum of our life experiences, our inner souls. An expressionless, perfectly smooth face is indeed lifeless—and therefore not really beautiful. Beauty is pretty features and good skin, but more than that, it is energy, enthusiasm, enjoyment, experience, a zest for life. Let it show on your face; it is what makes you you.

Occasional Changes and Your Skin

Skin and the Sun

It's like love and marriage—the two seem to be inseparable, but they're not always compatible. Should I merely add my voice to the chorus of "Stay out of the sun! It's only bad for you! Stay inside and close the shutters!"? That's unrealistic—it's hard to convince many people that the sun is poisonous for them since they look so fabulous in a tan! How many eighteen-year-olds—tanned and brown and gorgeous eighteen-year-olds—will believe me when I tell them that in ten or fifteen years, their skin will look like leather, their eyes will be wrinkled, and their faces will look ten years older than their age. So for those of us who will not stay indoors forever (and I am in this group, believe me), here are some things we should all know.

It is a fact that damage from the sun is cumulative. It doesn't happen in one day, nor does it happen in a week. But it will happen, because once you expose your skin to the sun over an extended period of time, the damage is irreversible. Those wrinkles will come —no doubt about it.

Taking careful care of your skin—throughout your life—nourishing it, moisturizing it, keeping it looking as beautiful as it can—is all for nought if you go out into the sun and dry it out making it flaky, spotted, wrinkled and perhaps cancerous. The price of a tan can be very high.

However, since it is unrealistic to expect us all to stay out of the sun forever, the best compromise may be the following:

• Go out into the sun, but do so before 10 A.M. and after 2 P.M., when the sun's rays are least dangerous.

• Wear a strong protective sun block, at least number 8 and preferably number 15 (there are even moisturizing sun blocks on the market); remember that wearing a sunscreen does not mean you won't get a tan—it simply means that you will block out the sun's harmful ultraviolet rays. Wearing a sun block means you will get no tan.

• Cover your head, and wear sunglasses at all times. Don't pick a pair just because they are fashionable and match your bathing suit. Pick out ones that are both attractive and have good lenses that will keep out the sun. (My motto is: Instead of getting six cheap pairs in one year—buy one of quality with optical lenses.)

• Another hint is to build up your suntan slowly, without burning the skin: The *melanin* in your body, which is a natural sunscreen, accumulates as you slowly tan.

• Perspiration is also a type of natural sunscreen—so when you play tennis in the sun, don't wipe off that sweat—instead, pat it down. But remember, when you come inside, cleanse your skin and moisturize it well. And don't use your sweat as an excuse not to wear a sun block. You need it to keep out those ultraviolet rays.

Please understand that I don't advocate giving up being outdoors, canceling all participation in sports, or banishing beach vacations, especially since moving around in the sun means you are not getting the amount of direct rays you would if you were lying on the sand getting fried. But I urge you to at least protect yourself from the sun. Get that sun block and use it. Also, be sure to drink a lot when you are in the sun—water, juices, iced tea—anything to replenish your supply of water. But don't drink too much alcohol, because when combined with the heat, alcohol drains you of energy and makes your heart beat faster. My rule is—for every piña colada, I drink two glasses of water.

Another no-no: Never put baby oil or any other oil on your skin and then go out into the sun. Take a look at a steak before you put oil on it for frying. Now fry it—see what happens to it? It shrivels up, all wrinkled and greasy. Would you want to kiss a fried steak? Think about it.

One added thought. If you have been a sun worshiper and you are now reading these ominous words—irreversible, damaging, wrinkles, dehydration—you've probably decided that it's too late to change. Besides, you look so great in a tan, and so awful without one—pale, face dry and lined—you may as well keep on getting tanned. This is a vicious cycle. Do yourself a favor—get out of it now. It's self-defeating. Stop the cycle, look directly into the mirror and take stock. Start caring for your skin immediately. Cleanse it, moisturize it—eat properly to plump out those lines. Treat the wrinkles to minimize the lines. Return to the sun, but protect your skin. Better now than never.

Water and Skin

I have spoken about moisturizing your skin with cream and about drinking water to moisturize it from the inside. In Chapter 7, Essential Luxuries, I will discuss bathing. Here are some other general hints about the relationship between your skin and water.

SWIMMING
Sea water can be therapeutic, but it is also drying. So after a swim in the ocean, rinse off the salt and reapply your sun block. After swimming in a chlorinated pool, it is important to shower to get the chlorine off your skin (I remove my suit in the shower, thus rinsing both the suit and myself in one stroke). Always lubricate the skin on your body and moisturize your face after swimming.

BATHING
As applicable to skin care, bathing is necessary to have clean skin. I believe baths are wonderful for relaxation, but for clean skin, showers are better. If you love baths, get into the habit of rinsing off afterward in the shower. When bathing I use the same soap on my body as I use on my face—because all my skin, from head to toe, is important. I keep a pumice stone in the tub to get rid of dead skin on my elbows and on the bottoms of my feet—two places many people forget. After a bath or shower, try rinsing with cool (not cold) water to close the pores all over your body, just as you do after a facial or a masque for your face. Consider your skin as one big sheet all over your body—it's all special, all fragile and it all needs care. Since it covers 100 percent of you, it needs almost that much attention.

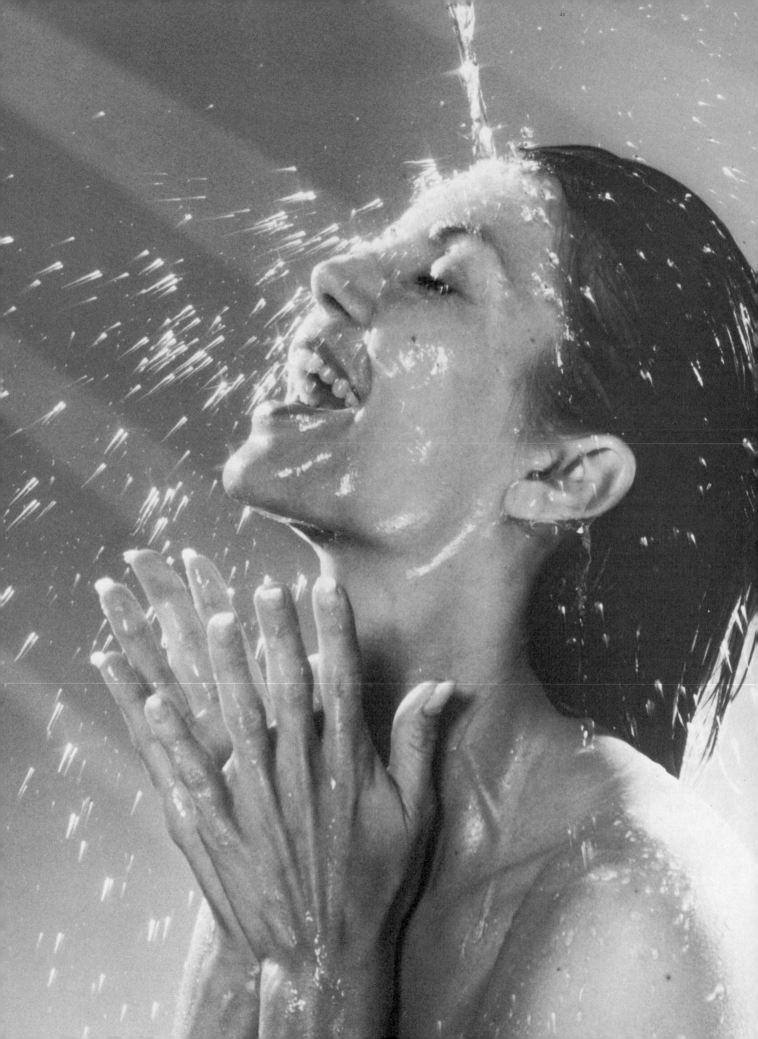

Changes in Climate

Changes in weather conditions definitely affect the condition of your skin and how you treat it. Depending on where you live, the weather changes when the seasons change, either minimally or drastically. Whatever the change, it is important to know how to take care of your skin in different climates. There are ways to make your skin not only survive the change of seasons but, by compensating for the changes, make sure it stays healthy.

IN COLD AND DRY WEATHER

In this climate you know you'll be frequently going from artificially heated homes to the cold and windy outdoors. The following hints will help you to cope with these sudden changes:

1. Never leave the house with moist skin or lips—you will have chapped skin almost instantly.

2. Drink as much water as you can to keep your skin moisturized from the inside. You can also increase your intake of oil in small amounts.

3. Moisturize your skin—if you have a heavier moisturizer on hand, use it. Use your eye cream, and a vitamin E stick on your lips (you can also use it under your eyes).

4. Protect your skin from the wind—wear a hat and gloves, and keep your face away from direct wind as much as possible. If you are skiing, consider wearing a ski mask.

5. If your home is heated by a radiator or forced-air heat, keep a humidifier or a glass of water in your bedroom to add moisture to the air.

6. Use a masque made of mayonnaise or honey, yogurt and egg yolk for added moisture.

7. Drink a hot beverage before you go out so your body will retain some of its heat after you go outdoors.

8. Don't sit in front of a heater or a fireplace and then go outdoors—the drastic change in temperature is bad for your skin.

IN COLD AND WET WEATHER

In this climate you face the same conditions as those listed above, except you don't need to worry as much about moisture. To deal with the cold, you'll need to:

1. Remember that because the cold keeps your pores closed, you will need to cleanse your skin dutifully to get at the dirt in them.

2. I use my moisturizer to minimize chapping of my skin, and a night cream to keep it moist while I sleep.

3. I use a lip balm, petroleum jelly and a vitamin E stick to keep my lips moist. In cold weather, we all have a tendency to breathe through our mouths, which results in moist lips turning into chapped lips. When I was filming in Chicago, I went through more lip balms than I had used in my entire life. But they were worth it!

4. Cold and wet weather can make your skin splotchy. To even it out, put a cucumber masque (blend some cucumbers with yogurt) or wet, cooled tea bags (with tannin) on your skin.

IN HOT AND DRY WEATHER

1. You need a thin moisturizer in hot and dry weather because you have to be wary of clogging up your pores—they need to be open so you can perspire. But if you feel your skin is getting dehydrated, use a night cream during the day. And apply it as often as you feel you need it.

2. I use an eye cream faithfully.

3. Drink as much as you can—again, perspiration is healthy but it will rid you of a lot of water that your body and your skin need. I alternate my water with iced tea.

4. Step up your intake of oil for added moisture. I take a tablespoon of mineral oil before I go to bed.

5. You may need some extra potassium in your system—eat bananas and broccoli.

6. Use a moisturizing masque twice as often as in other climates —try making one with honey, avocado and mustard in equal

—try making one with honey, avocado and mustard in equal amounts. You can also make one with one tablespoon of mayonnaise, one tablespoon of honey and an egg yolk. Follow the instructions for applying a masque on page 47.

7. Use a humidifier at home or keep a bowl or glass of water in the room(s).

IN HOT AND HUMID, SOMETIMES WINDY WEATHER

Dallas. In July and August. I know this one very well. Every year we film in Dallas in the summer months, when it is very hot and very humid, and every year my skin rebels. By now I know that I have to take care of my skin more at this time than at others.

1. In summer, the heat stimulates the oil glands: They secrete more, so your face is oilier. I know that I have to keep my pores as clean as possible at this time, and be sure to close them with cold water or ice.

2. I wear sun block under my makeup to be sure the sun won't damage my face. We shoot outdoors, and people who live in this climate by necessity spend a lot of time outdoors; so the rule in Dallas is that sun block or, at the very least, a sunscreen, is essential.

3. I try not to touch my face during the day. The wind always brings dirt and dust, and because it is so hot and humid, these impurities stick to the skin on my hands and on my face. So I cover or shield my face as much as possible.

4. I make sure to keep my cleansing sponges and buffs extra clean because bacteria grow in the heat.

5. I use an astringent during the day to clean the grease off my face and help keep my pores closed.

6. If I am not shooting, I wear very light makeup so I am clogging my skin as little as possible.

7. I use a commercial honey-almond face scrub four times a week. It cleans all the ''garbage'' out of my beleaguered skin.

8. I give myself a facial once a week to both clean and moisturize my skin.

9. I use an eye cream at night and under my eye makeup,

because in this weather, even with sunglasses, people squint, and squinting gives us all wrinkles.

10. I drink a lot of water, and eat salt (which I *never* do in other climates) because perspiration results in a loss of sodium which the body needs. A word here about perspiration: It is a necessary cooling system in the body—it is important to perspire. Wearing a deodorant should only minimize odor, not prevent perspiration. So it is important to keep those pores clean—or they will clog up and your ability to perspire normally will be hampered.

Travel and Your Skin

The above hints on dealing with your skin in different climates apply not only to where you live but where you travel. Since travel often takes us to places with varying weather conditions, all of the preceding hints may be applicable to trips we may take at one time or another.

But traveling also demands other plans. On pages 122 to 127 I discuss The Perfect Makeup Bag. For traveling it is also necessary to take along your skin care products. I keep sample sizes of each of my creams—moisturizer, eye cream, baby oil (which can also serve as a makeup remover), soap, astringent, cleanser and brush, and a scrub—so when I travel I can use the same products I always use, without having to pack and carry large jars and bottles. If you don't have sample sizes of your products, put a little of each in small plastic bottles made for traveling and label them (or mark them with different colors of nail polish) so you will always know which cream is which.

I also carry an atomizer of water and one of perfume, a hand cream (perfect for use on an airplane when my skin gets so dry), a tube of Aloe Vera gel (great for skin care and emergency burns), a tube of petroleum jelly (a good lip gloss and moisturizer) and a drying stick for those unwelcome pimples and blemishes.

Since I fly on a lot of airplanes, I have also developed ways to take care of my skin while flying. The perfect way to fly would be to get on an airplane with no makeup on—only moisturizer on the skin so it will not get dehydrated in the cabin air. But for most women this is unrealistic—for whatever reasons, we want to look attractive on the airplane. Thus, I make up my face basically as I do every morning (see Chapter 3), except that I put on more moisturizer under my eyes and less makeup everywhere—everything is applied with a lighter touch to let my skin breathe.

I have learned through experience that on an airplane skin dehydrates and absorbs makeup. So I keep an atomizer filled with water to occasionally spray my face, and I touch up my makeup at the end of the flight. I also do my "drink a lot of water" routine—and the flight attendants are never surprised—because they know better than anyone the toll that airplane travel takes on the skin.

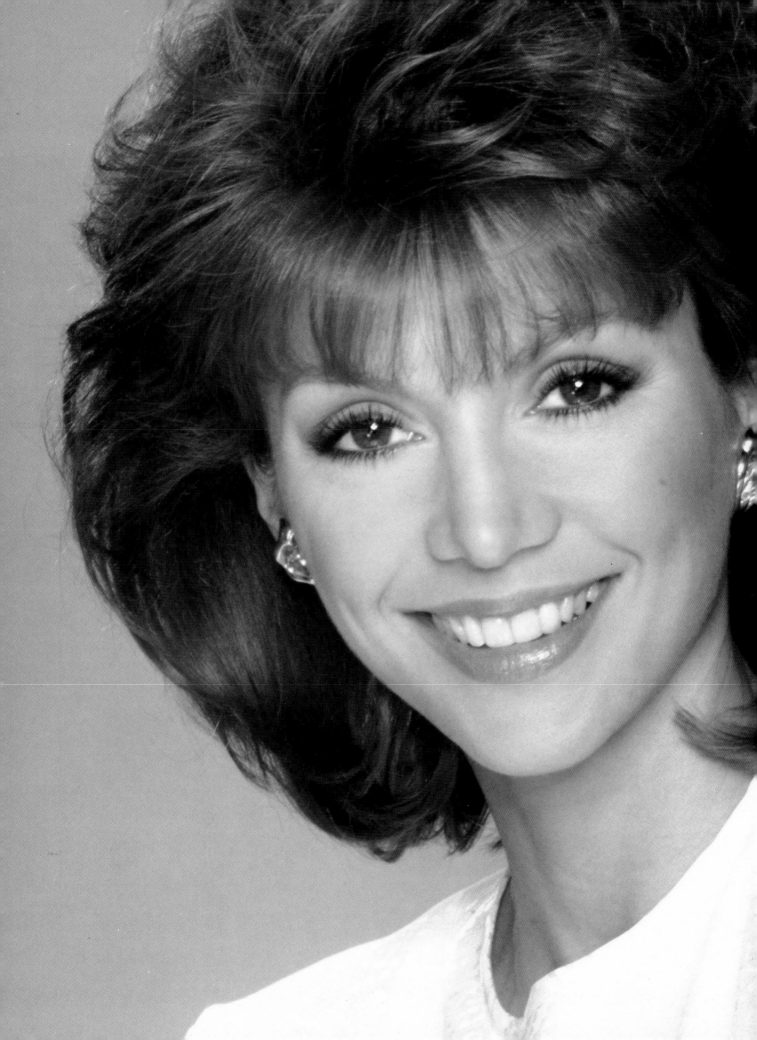

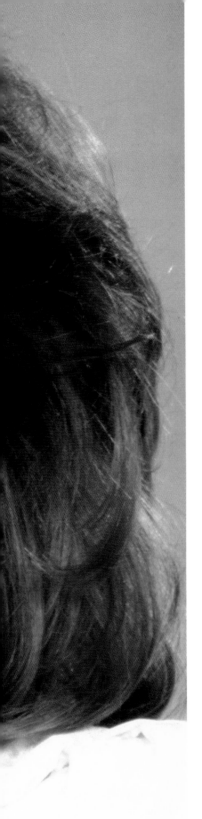

CHAPTER 3

THE FINAL TOUCH: MAKEUP

I have never considered myself a raving beauty.

That does not mean I don't like the way I look; it does not mean I don't like myself. It does not mean that Victoria Principal as Pam in "Dallas," or in photographs, or in magazines, or in everyday life is not attractive. But I get there, as I said, with a little help from my friends: the foundation, the mascara, the lipstick, the blush, the powder—all combine in a special and deliberate way to disguise the less-than-perfect features and to make the best of what I have.

And when I come home, when the cameras are gone, when the lights go out, when dinner is over, and the makeup comes off, there is me. Not so different from that other lady, except the skin is somewhat sallow, the eyes a little tired, the skin a little dry. Under the makeup, it's still me. And I like that me because I am the same person with or without any makeup.

The funny thing is, people often look at me and tell me how pretty I look without makeup (now I'm not talking about times when I have an obviously made-up nighttime face, or the one I get photographed in, but my "natural" everyday face). What they don't realize is that I do have makeup on, but it's so natural and subtle that it's not noticeable. That is because a well-made-up everyday face is a face that doesn't look made up. And that is deliberate.

This everyday face is not an accident. There is a reason for every shadow, every brush stroke, every line. The method is calculated, but the result looks natural. That is the secret of the perfectly made-up face—it doesn't hide the person underneath, the person inside. It doesn't lie about me. The makeup doesn't hide me just as it would not hide you. I don't use it as a mask. What you are is what you get —but the made-up version is prettier to the eye.

Just ask anyone on the set of "Dallas" who has seen me at five in the morning without a stitch of makeup on my face, only my moisturizer. This is not what you call a perfectly beautiful face. Believe me, I know! I don't delude myself. What my friends do notice when I have makeup on is the face that is made up, not the makeup itself. That is the key—to notice and react to the total picture, the painted canvas, if you will, without noticing the brush strokes, the layers that went into creating the final look, the shadows and the colors, the careful planning and work it all took.

This is true for any face. We are all a little plainer when we are bare, and we can all be lovelier with makeup. Of course, it is your choice. But any woman can, with makeup applied properly, be it a minimal natural touch or a more complicated look, enhance her own beauty. It is not difficult; it is quite simple. It is not time-consuming; it is surprisingly quick. It is not false; it can be flatteringly natural.

Putting on makeup is like being an artist. But unlike the artist, you don't start with a perfect canvas. If you really look at a woman you consider to be "perfectly" beautiful, chances are you will find that her features are not perfect at all, that what she has done is made the most of what she has by accentuating her best features and turning those imperfections, those irregularities, into pluses.

Most of the time I wear makeup simply to make *me* look better, to give me more confidence in my appearance. At other times, when I am not at my best, I use it to look and feel better. And sometimes I wear it to be noticed, to stand out in a crowd.

We all have such moments in our lives—when we want to create a stir, to be the center of attention. These occasional reasons are perfectly healthy, and there are ways to use makeup effectively to create all these effects.

Don't try to look like anyone else, because you can never really succeed. At the end of each evening, you are going to have to wash off that face and come to terms with the person who looks back at you in the mirror. That is the real you. This doesn't mean you can't learn how to wear makeup from other people. But I have always believed that women kid themselves when they think they can make themselves look like someone else and that no one will notice, or see through the charade.

Everyone has her own ideal sense of beauty. There came a point in my life when I came to terms with the fact that I was never going to be a blond, blue-eyed lanky beauty. As you can see by my early photographs, my face started out round, and I tried very hard to make it oval; that was my idea of beauty. Then, as I lost my baby fat my face became heart shaped. I realized that not only was my face heart shaped, but that I liked it that way, and that I was not only *not* going to make up my face to hide this and other characteristics, I was going to accentuate them.

Makeup should be the added touch that makes the best of what is you and you alone, not the tool to make you look like someone you are not. It is not only unfair to yourself if you try to resemble someone else—it will be obvious to everyone around you. It would be sad to never see yourself as you are, and sadder still to spend your life trying to look like some ideal in a magazine or on TV. It is futile, particularly since that person out there has used makeup in a certain way to create an illusion specifically for the cameras, not for real life.

There is a great difference between the makeup I wear every day and what I wear when I am in front of the camera. What I do with my professional face in terms of molding and sculpting my features is much more complex than what I do for my everyday face. It's done because the camera looks at my face differently than you would in life. Because of my profession, I will wear at least four or five times as much makeup in my lifetime as other women (this is not great news for my skin, which is why I pay such careful attention to it).

But the point is that the people you see on television and in magazines are wearing makeup that is not comparable with the makeup *they* wear in their "real" lives. There is an unreality in photographs and in films that cannot and should not be translated into real life.

It would also be tragic to use makeup as a mask behind which you can hide. Now it may be perfectly fine to put on a mask for one night, to be noticed, to call attention to yourself, as long as you know that is what you are doing. It is another thing, however, to pretend to be someone else, using the makeup as a shield behind which you feel more safe.

Part of coming to terms with your makeup ceremony, your makeup attitude, is really seeing who you are. Look in that mirror and see your face as if it were the face of a stranger. Take note of those things you immediately like. You may be surprised when you like something you always thought of as less than perfect. Now, rather than hiding it, you can take advantage of it—it is yours and yours alone. It is what makes you unique. For example, for years I tried to deny I have almond-shaped eyes. Don't ask me why—I just believed that round eyes were "perfect," so I developed a way, by using pencils, liners, shadows and blushes, to turn my almond-shaped eyes into round ones. But I, too, have come a long way. I have come to understand that my features are my own, and I have learned how, with makeup, I can make them work for me.

I also learned that makeup is most effective when it reflects my energy, my enthusiasm, my personality. It is important to understand your personality and your own life style so that you can wear a makeup that fits it and doesn't look out of place. If you are a private person who leads a casual life, there is no need for you to put on a flamboyant face every morning. It's not you. On the other hand, if you are an outgoing, social person who leads an active life that brings you in contact with other people, a bare face may not work for you and you may want to have a more noticeable look. There are times when you may want to be showy—and there are ways to achieve that. But as a rule, for your everyday life, you must be true to yourself and wear makeup that goes with your personality and life. Your makeup should mesh with you, not clash with you.

Just as it is important to keep in perspective what makeup can and should do for you, so it is wise to understand the importance of finding a makeup that will work to help you look your best. This doesn't mean that once you choose a makeup that flatters you you have to keep it for the rest of your life. I certainly don't advocate getting a look that suits you and staying with it for the next forty years. You can periodically update your look as times and styles change. But I am against being consumed by fads in cosmetic products and in how to use them.

I believe that as consumers we need to carefully decide for ourselves what looks good on us. (We ought to have some say in the matter—American consumers spend over $4 *billion* a year on makeup!) I love to try some of the new makeup shades and techniques, but as a rule, I stay away from extremes. Thus, when a few years ago everything around me was purple, I must admit I was tempted to purple-ize myself. But not for long—when I tried purple blusher, I looked like a Halloween victim. I tried the new fad—and realized it was not for me. But the trip to the cosmetic counter was not in vain; I found a new shade of tawny blush that was somewhat brighter than the one I had been using, and loved it! And it was the *right* shade. It complimented my foundation, my skin color and the color of my hair. And I looked much better than I did in the purple.

The lesson I learned is that each of us needs to find a *basic* look that suits us, that enhances our own individual features and melds with our own personalities. Then, as styles change or new trends come about, we will know how to discriminate between a product or a technique that suits our particular makeup look.

Actually the makeup industry has come a long way since the days when Egyptian women used berries for color and white chalk for foundation. Many of today's products have nourishing compounds in them; the color variations are almost limitless; the tools make both simple and sophisticated applications easier and more efficient; and the tools and techniques that makeup artists have developed over the years make us more beautiful.

THE PRINCIPLES OF MAKEUP

The Tools

In order to put makeup on correctly, you need the right tools. These tools are simple, inexpensive, usually unbreakable and easy to keep clean, and you can get them at almost any supermarket, beauty supply store, five and dime, or drugstore in your neighborhood. Here is the basic list:

• *Flat, round makeup sponge:* This is the sponge with which I put the foundation on my face (before I blend it with my fingertips). Wash it out with your hand soap after use each and every time. If you do, it should last you about two weeks.

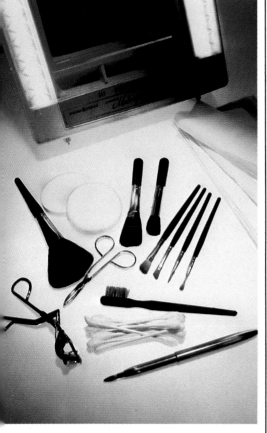

• *Flat powder puff:* Get the cheapest kind you can find, because these are perishable and should not be used more than three or four times. This is to use with your translucent powder, usually in the evening because it will set the makeup better. (During the day it is better to apply your powder with a brush, because it gives a lighter look.)

• *Set of brushes:* These can last for a long time, so splurge and get good ones with sable hairs. Brushes are now sold in sets (for six to fifteen dollars a set), which can include two blush brushes, an eyebrow brush (you can also use it to separate your lashes when they stick together), an eyelash brush, an eye shadow brush, and sometimes brushes with which you apply eye liner. This set is a terrific long-term investment, without which you really cannot have an efficient and workable makeup routine. If you find that you like applying translucent powder with a brush, buy the largest one you can find. Note that you must take care of these brushes—just put them in a sink full of shampoo (if it is good enough for your hair, it is good enough for your brushes!) and rinse well. Lay them out on a towel on your counter, and let them dry. Do this once a week and they will last for years.

• *Lipstick brush* (the retractable is the best kind): Personally, since they invented the lipstick pencil, I have done away with using the lipstick brush. But if you use tube lipstick, this brush is a must.

• *Eyebrow tweezers*

• *Eyelash curler*

• *Tissues and/or cotton balls or pads and cotton swabs:* You use them to remove and blot makeup. I prefer to use tissues to remove and pat down makeup. You can keep cotton balls or pads in a jar on your makeup table. If you wear contact lenses, be aware that the balls or pads can fuzz in your eyes.

• *Makeup mirror*—preferably with proper lights (see page 121).

Now that's not a lot of equipment, is it? The rest is done with your fingertips.

The Products

For a complete makeup routine (I assume you already have all your skin care products), you will need the following cosmetics (you may not use each of these products every day, but you should have them on hand).

- Moisturizer

- Undereye concealer—to match your skin color

- Foundation—three shades: (1) matching your skin; (2) lighter than your skin (highlighter—optional); (3) three shades darker than your skin (contour—optional)

- Cream blush

- Powder blush

- Translucent powder

- Eye shadows—preferably powder

- Eye liner pencil

- Mascara

- Eyebrow pencil (optional)

- Lip liner pencil (optional)

- Lip gloss/lipstick

The Terms

Before you learn how to put on makeup, you need to know what the products are, what they can and cannot do and how best to use them. A few definitions will help you get started.

CONCEALER

A concealer is used to hide undereye circles. Choose a concealer close to the color of your skin; they usually come in three colors—light, medium and dark (whatever color you choose, make sure it is close to your skin color—and don't get white! That will result in your not only looking like an owl, but will actually accentuate the circles by making them very noticeable). There are some concealers with other colors in them, which is useful for certain kinds of dark circles (for example, if you have very dark blue circles under your eyes, get a concealer with a touch of green in it). Whenever I use a concealer I make sure it is about three shades lighter than my regular foundation, because I then blend it with my foundation. Choosing the color of a concealer is personal, as long as you leave out that white.

The easiest concealers to apply are those in a wand because they are so creamy they can be applied smoothly, without stretching or pulling the skin (the skin under your eyes is very sensitive and can be stretched easily). Concealers that come in a small pot require you to dip your finger in them, something that is difficult to do if you have long nails (so use the outside tip of your nail).

You may now ask, what is the difference between a concealer cream and a highlighter? A highlighter is a brighter cream that is made specifically to attract light, and will thus stand out more than your concealer, which is made to be blended and to disappear.

FOUNDATION

The word foundation means exactly that: It is the foundation, the basis, of your makeup routine. If it isn't right, your whole look may be off. Foundations are either oil or water based. Some skin experts will tell you that if you have oily skin, you should use a water-based foundation, and if you have dry skin, use an oil-based one. The skin expert I trust most, Aida Thibiant, says that most of the women she cares for have skin that is both dry and oily—combination skin—and for all these women, a water-based foundation is best. Moreover, a water-based foundation prevents the makeup's penetration into the skin.

It is important to choose a foundation similar in color to your own skin. This is really easy—it is a matter of trial and error, and will take at the most an hour of your time in a department store or makeup center. Here you can test different shades of foundation and other products to find the right one for you. Don't try the first shade of foundation and say, "Okay, I'll take it." Try one color on the inside of your wrist (never on your face—that is a good way to spread bacteria) and walk around for a few minutes. Now look at the shade again, and then try another one. It is well worth the time to find a foundation that will look good on you.

If you think you will be interested in contouring and or highlighting your features, you need to buy another foundation a shade lighter than the one that matches your skin, and one that is three shades darker than your basic color. Again, a good cosmetician or a sales-person in a cosmetics department can help you choose the colors you will need.

PRIMER

I don't use a primer, but I think it may be a good idea for some women. Under-makeup primer temporarily evens out the color of your skin when used under your foundation. If, for example, your skin is ruddy or quite sallow (or when you have the beginnings of a tan and your skin seems splotchy in different areas of your face), you can take the primer and spread it all over your face to make your complexion more evenly colored. Be careful not to put on too much primer, because if you do, by the time you add foundation to your face you will look as if you have on too much makeup.

This is a good product that can help any skin discoloration or blotchiness.

HIGHLIGHTER

This is a special cream that attracts light and is used in conjunction with contouring cream to sculpt a face to minimize and maximize selected features. It is a cosmetic that creates illusions. A light foundation can be used for the same purpose.

CONTOURING

Contouring is an option which I would guess many of you will choose not to undertake because not only can it be difficult and unsightly if done incorrectly, but also because many women don't really need to contour their faces.

If not done properly, contouring can and will make your face look dirty. Believe me—I've been there. The first time I used a contour cream I looked as if some child had painted two brown lines on the sides of my face. The next time I looked as if I forgot to wash my face. Another time it seemed to me that when I was finished applying the dark cream, my face resembled a connect-the-dot picture. *Contouring takes practice!* It is not meant to be noticed but rather to define or conceal. You don't use it like a foundation or a hand cream —you can't just throw it on and leave it there. It must be delicately and precisely placed, and then forgotten. If someone notices you have contoured your face, you did it wrong!

What contouring does is make the best of the attractive features on your face and minimize those that are not as pleasing. It works on the principle that light refracts and dark absorbs light. So whenever you use a contour cream (or a dark foundation) you are going to be shadowing those features. When you use a highlighter to lighten, or refract the light that hits your face, you will be punching out, or calling attention to, that feature.

Here is another way to explain it. Light maximizes and dark deemphasizes, or minimizes, a feature. So if you have a nose you consider to be too wide for your face (like mine is), put contour cream down either side of the nose, put highlighter down the front, and you will have made your nose look narrower. You have created an optical illusion that your nose is not wide but narrow. For other problems contouring can solve, see page 115.

The most important lesson to be learned when using contouring is that it must be blended. When you blend the dark cream with your foundation, so there is no visible dividing line between the two, you will be surprised at how effective the illusion is. The dark cream literally disappears, and the result is a redefined feature.

When it comes to choosing a contouring cream, it is important to pick a shade that will work with your own particular skin type (remember that contouring cream by nature is some shade of brown). A contour cream should complement both your foundation and the color of your skin. For example, I have a *light olive complexion,* almost Oriental. I have found that a contour cream several shades darker than my skin with some taupe in it is perfect for me. Let's say you have a *ruddy complexion* and you are using a foundation that has some green in it. You will then want to choose a contouring cream that is brown with a green cast to it. For a fair-haired person with *light skin,* a contour that has the essence of rose or pink in it will work well. For *dark-skinned* women (dark olive), you will probably want to use a darker tawny brown that won't turn orange on you. The same will hold true for a black skin.

The best advice about choosing a contour cream is to find a saleswoman at a cosmetics counter who seems to know what contouring is and can help you choose the right one for you. With contouring, it is so important that the color suit you (and that you apply it correctly), that it is worth your while to spend the time at the store to find the appropriate product.

BLUSH

There are many different kinds of blush (sometimes known as rouge, but I love the word blush because the way you apply the color is to give the impression that you are blushing, that you have a flush of color). Blush comes in powder, liquid or cream. I prefer a water-based cream blush for the first application in the morning, and the powder blush for re-touching during the day, because the cream blush goes on smoothly, is absorbed nicely into your skin, and will last for some time, and you can put powder blush over it anytime during the day. If you start out your day with powder blush, you cannot retouch with the cream because it will cake and/or blotch on your face. Also, if you apply powder blush on skin that has only foundation on it, it may splotch—the moisture in your skin will grab it in different places and it will be so spotty, chances are you'll have to start all over again. Powder blush is most effective over a foundation and cream blush on an already powdered face.

As far as color is concerned, I have found that the best idea is to have one blush you can wear almost anytime and with everything. This is a blush that compliments your skin tone and is in the color range of your skin. When choosing the cream blush and the powder blush, make sure that the cream is a shade darker than the powder because it will be absorbed into your skin and may come down a shade or two, whereas the powder blush will sit on your skin and hold its color.

POWDER

There are basically two kinds of face powder: One is a translucent powder which is loose and applied with a large brush; the other is pressed, comes in a compact and is applied with a small puff. The purpose of using powder is to set your makeup. It may seem as if, by applying the powder, you will be messing up what you have carefully applied, but this is not so. Powder really fixes it in place, and, contrary to popular opinion, does not clog your skin. Surprisingly, powder has some other beneficial effects. One is that it protects your skin from the elements in the air. Another is that it absorbs extra oil on your skin (this is good news for those of you with spots of oily skin on your face, something almost all of us have).

Many women choose powders with different colors in them (some have essence of green, others purple and still others red or copper). I prefer to leave the color for the blush. I always use a powder similar in color to my skin and/or my foundation. I also stay away from baby powders—they belong on babies' bottoms or on your body after a bath. Using baby powder as face powder can give your skin a white, pallid look.

EYE SHADOW

This is a cream or a powder that comes in many colors and textures and is used to accentuate your eyes. I prefer powder shadows because it is easier to control the application with a brush. It is a good idea to start with a neutral beige shadow, a brown one, a pink one and a dark purple. These are fairly neutral tones that will look natural and enhance any eyes.

EYE PENCIL

An eye pencil is used in the crease of the lid or as an eye liner. Eye pencils come in many colors, and the newest are creamy enough to spread like cream eye shadow. Used with shadow, pencils can effectively compliment your eyes.

An eyebrow pencil is harder and is made to be used on the eyebrows.

MASCARA

There are several kinds of mascara to choose from. Cake mascara is popular with models, because it lasts a long time. I think you can get an equally effective look with the tube mascara. There is waterproof mascara, which is fine if you swim or cry a lot; it stays intact on your lashes and will only come off with an eye makeup remover specifically made for this type of mascara. Regular mascara or water-soluble mascara will run if you tear and is easily removed with plain old water. Yet another kind of mascara has little fibers in it to make your lashes look thicker. However, you should know that the fibers can get into your eyes, so be extra careful when you use it, particularly if you wear contact lenses. As far as the color of mascara goes, I advocate using black for everyone except blondes, who often look better in a brown-black or dark brown mascara. Mascaras also come in blue, green, even red. I truly prefer to stick to the browns and blacks for the most natural look.

LIPSTICK AND LIP GLOSS

These are creams that should only be used on the lips. Lipstick usually comes in a tube and can be applied directly to the lips. I prefer, however, to use a *lipstick brush* which touches the lipstick and can then be applied to your lips (it gives you more control). I also use a *lip liner pencil* to outline my lips before I apply the lipstick.

Lip gloss comes in a wand, a tube, or a pot, and is creamy and translucent. It is often worn alone, or sometimes over lipstick to give your lips additional shine. For more information on lips, see pages 106 to 109.

THE STEPS OF MAKING UP

The process of putting on makeup must always start with clean skin. There is no point in putting makeup on skin that already has yesterday's makeup on it—first because you will only clog up your pores and hurt your skin, and second because the makeup will cake and blotch and may look strange and unflattering on last night's leftovers. So, please, don't carry your face over from day to day.

It is morning. You are awake; you have done your stretch exercises, taken a shower and started your circulation going (thus you have some color in your face). You have gone through your cleansing routine, ending up with your astringent, and have patted your moisturizer gently into your skin. (Remember, that means moisturizing eye cream under and around the eyes, and your facial moisturizer on your face.)

That done, you are ready for the makeup routine. As you are getting used to this routine (and especially as you are reading this) it may seem that it will take forever. Don't be discouraged. It won't. Following are three basic morning makeup routines you can choose from, depending on your life style, your plans for the day and your mood. Both the two- and five-minute routines are easy and require little explanation. When I describe the ten-minute routine, I will discuss each step in greater detail, so even if you end up using only the two- or five-minute routine, read the ten-minute one to find out my many tips for the effective and attractive application of makeup.

The Two-Minute Makeup Routine (Or the Pared-Down Look, or the No-Bother Face)

There is really no such thing as an honest-to-goodness, no-bother face. If there are only two things you want to do to make yourself presentable to go out, wear a dark hat and sunglasses. There is, however, a minimal, two-minute makeup routine that I have found adequate for some days. Please remember that you really are the best judge of what you need and want to do and what looks best on you. So you decide what you want to use and what options you want to leave out.

Assuming you have taken care of your skin, that it is clean, that you used your astringent and your moisturizer, you have the following choices (pick whatever things you want to do to your face):

1. If you have circles under your eyes, you will need to put a dab of concealer or your lightest foundation under your eyes, and blend well.

2. Now put a dot of your foundation on each eyelid, and blend again.

3. Take your cream blusher, and put under each cheekbone, and blend.

4. Curl your eyelashes with the eyelash curler, and apply one coat of mascara.

5. Dab on sheer lipstick or a little lip gloss.

6. If you have the time and the inclination, apply a second coat of mascara to your lashes, and you are done.

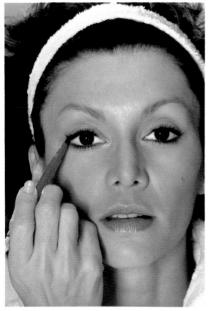

The Five-Minute Makeup Routine

1. Blend the concealer under your eyes.

2. Dot your regular foundation with a sponge on your cheeks, forehead, eyes, nose and chin, and blend gently with your fingertips. Don't stretch the skin by pulling it!

3. Use your cream blush along the cheekbones, and blend.

4. Put a touch of beige powder eye shadow on your eyelids (this is optional).

5. Take black eye pencil, dip it in your mascara, and draw a fine line between and in your upper eyelashes. This will open up your eyes and will last all day. Use the same pencil on the lower lid (no mascara this time) and smudge the line with a cotton swab.

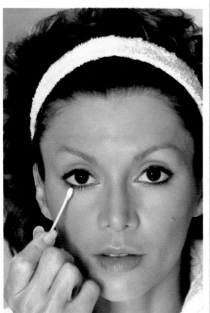

6. Curl your eyelashes with your curler (hold to a count of ten). Put on a layer of mascara.

7. Brush translucent powder all over your face to set the makeup.

8. Put another layer of mascara on your lashes.

9. Put lip gloss or your lipstick on your lips.

The Ten-Minute Makeup Routine

I love this routine. It took practice, trial and error, and a lot of listening and learning to get it down right. Here, then, complete with little tidbits here and there, is my very own makeup routine that will work for anyone. (For extra tips that depend on the shape of your face, the color of your complexion and the size and shape of your eyes and lips, see Types of Complexions and Features, pages 96 to 109.

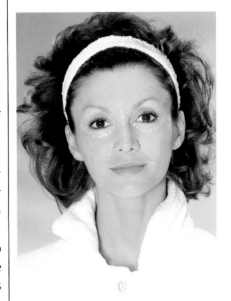

1. Most women need to put some concealer under their eyes to cover up shadows or so-called "dark circles." The reasons for these shadows are varied. For some women, they are hereditary; for others it's a sign of sinus problems (see a doctor); and for still others it's as simple as needing more sleep.

I use a wand-type concealer three shades lighter than my regular foundation, dotting it under my eyes, down my nose (to highlight for daytime use), and in the "smile" creases from my nose to my lips. Then I blend carefully.

If you use a cream concealer in a pot, put a dab of cream on one fingertip. Now pat it gently under your eyes, then pat with the tips of your fingers to smooth it out. *Never, ever* stretch the skin under the eyes—it will stretch with time by itself, and doesn't need any help from you. Pat gently at all times.

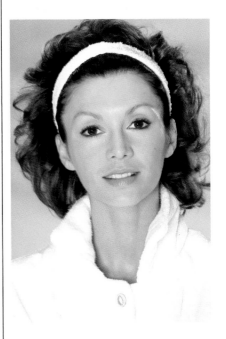

1

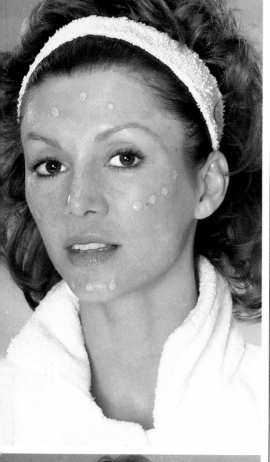

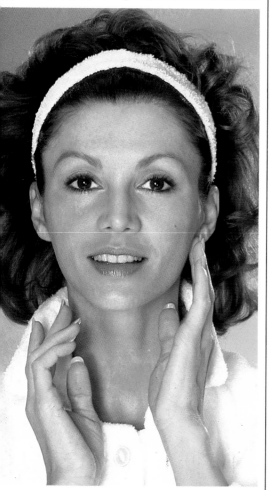

2. I have three shades of foundation. One matches my skin color and is used for overall coverage. Another is a shade lighter than my skin (for me that is ivory, quite a light color) which is used for lightening and highlighting certain parts of my face. The third is darker than my skin color and is used for contouring other parts of my face. This sounds complicated, so take a breath and take this in (for most people, one shade of foundation—the one that matches the color of your skin—is enough).

On a regular nonworking day, I put on the foundation closest to the color of my skin (you can get a foundation with a touch of pink or peach in it—some are made to compensate for the lack of color in your skin). My foundation is water based, which I think is the best kind, because it clogs the pores less than oil-based foundations. I put a dab of the foundation on my dry sponge, then pat it on my cheeks, my forehead, my eyelids (or you can use a product made to set eye makeup), my chin and under it, my nose and right up to my hairline. You can even put a dab on each earlobe.

Then with light strokes (never stretching or pulling—your skin is fragile, so treat it gently!) with my clean fingertips, I blend the foundation all over my face to make it look as natural as possible. Remember, this is not paint I am putting on. Foundation should look like one continuous color—no streaks or lines anywhere. The secret to applying it well is to layer it. I put on a little at a time and blend it into my skin. I want to be able to see my skin through the foundation. If I feel I need more coverage, I can always add more foundation only in the spots where it seems to be missing. You don't need to put another layer all over your face. Remember, taking off the extra foundation you carelessly slobbered on is hard to do. The secret of applying makeup is doing it a little at a time and blending it well.

By this time the heat of my body has warmed up my skin and the foundation goes on smoothly. I continue to pat and blend, never rubbing or stretching (dab gently now and your future skin will be in great shape), making sure it goes near (but not into) my hairline, and over my chin line. Nothing is worse than seeing a line of makeup ending at the chin. Also remember that your makeup will be noticeable if you don't blend it up to the hairline at the ear.

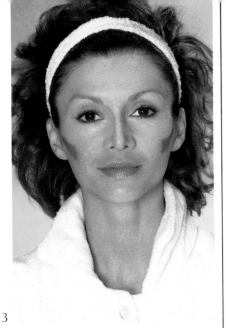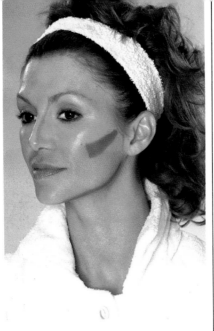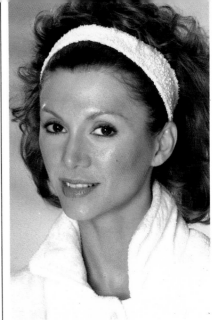

3

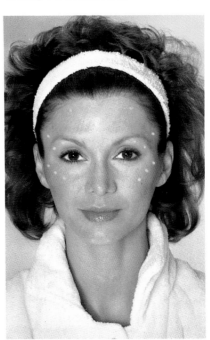

3. Most people do not need to contour their faces for daytime wear. But, if you have a nose you'd like to look thinner, or you want to contour some other feature, this is the time to do it, before you put on any more makeup. For example, to make your nose look thinner, take your darker shade of foundation (mine is a taupy brown) and shade your nose on either side. Blend the shadow with your fingertips so there is no line showing. Now take your highlighter on your fingertip, make a line running down the front of your nose and blend. When you are done you should be able to see nothing, except a thinner nose. If you have two dark lines on either side of your nose, chances are you put on too much contour. Always start by putting on a little at a time, and blend.

4. Now it's time for the blusher. I always start with a cream blush because if you want more color later, you can always brush on your powder blush. If you put on powder blush first, over your foundation, it may cake. As for using only powder blush—I think a cream blush gives me a better foundation of color that seems to last longer on my skin. I put the cream blush on my fingertips, then pat it onto my cheekbones, and place a dab on my forehead (I apply it just at my hairline at the top of my forehead, then across the width of my hairline, leaving it about one-quarter inch from either side). Now it goes on the tip of my nose (it makes me look healthy—almost as if I've been exposed to a little sun and gotten a bit of color from it). Then I put a dot on the tip of my chin and I blend so that it doesn't just look like a round circle but rather like a glow of health. I pat it down, not stretching the skin, until it is blended in. I put some under my eyebrows, just under the far end of the brow itself, because it gives me a wonderful feeling of depth. Now, as I look in the mirror, I see that I have a glow to my face.

4

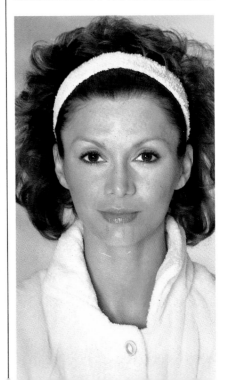

5

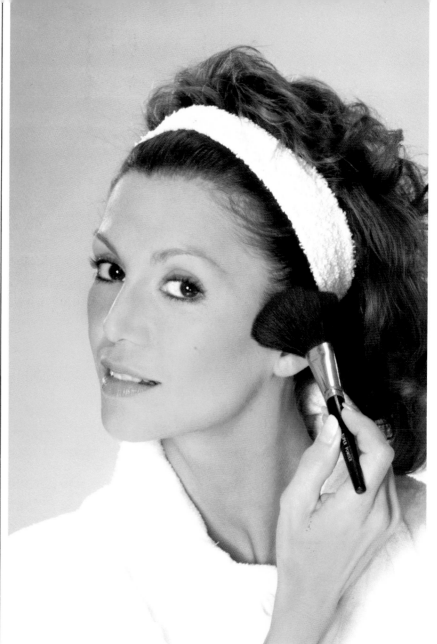

6

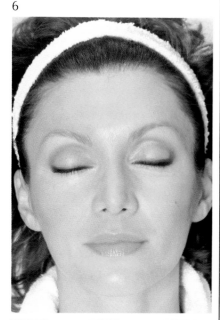

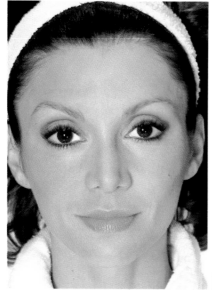

5. Now take your loose translucent powder and the powder brush (this should be the largest in your collection of brushes) and brush your whole face lightly to set your makeup. Please remember how I feel about baby powder—it belongs on a baby. Use a translucent powder for your face so it will fix in place the makeup you have worked so hard to create. (And just before you are ready to leave your house, you may want to add another brush of powder; then take your atomizer filled with water and spray your face. No, this won't mess up all your hard work. It will set your makeup for the whole day, and make your face look dewy and soft.)

6. I now take my neutral tone of powder eye shadow (beige, taupe, soft pink, gray, or muted mauve) and lightly brush it over my lids, under my brows and a touch in the crease above the eye. That's it for shadow for daytime wear.

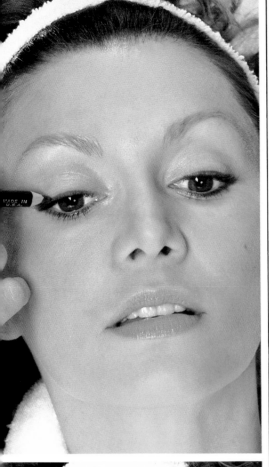

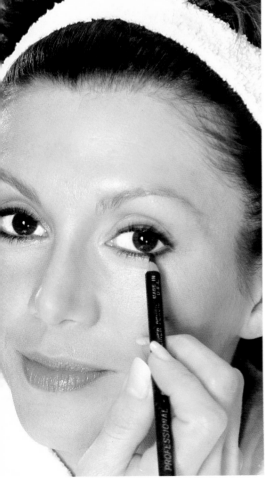

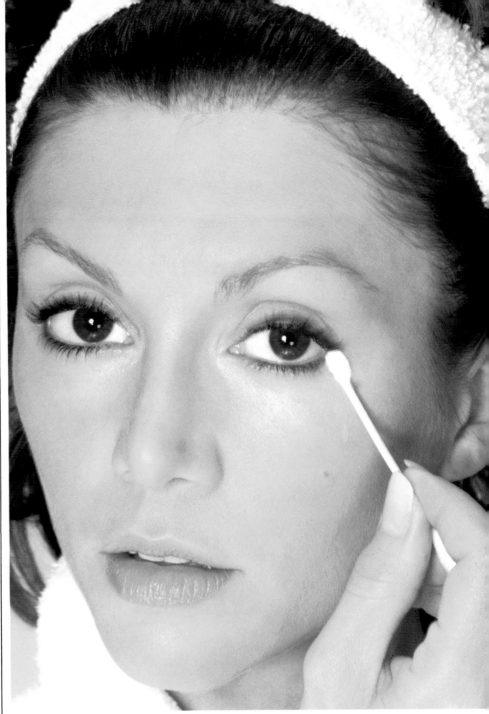

7

7. Now I take my eye pencil, dip it into the mascara and use it to line my eye on the top lid, between each lash as in the five-minute makeup routine. Then I draw a soft line (without dipping the pencil into the mascara) along the lash line of my upper lid and just below the lash line of the lower lid. Then gently smudge the upper and bottom lines with a cotton swab to soften them.

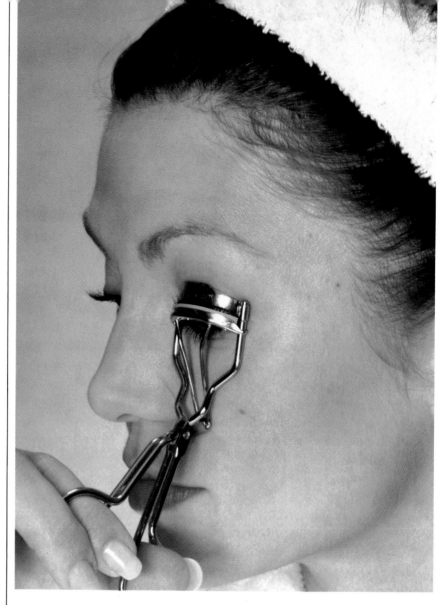

8

8. The magic touch—mascara. When God invented mascara, She did a good thing. Mascara is the single thing (besides a good foundation) that makes your face glow by making your eyes sparkle. I never go without it.

The first step is to use your eyelash curler—*never* ever put on mascara and then curl your lashes. They will fall out, stick to the curler and damage the follicles. So always curl your eyelashes first (unless you have naturally curly eyelashes, in which case I envy you).

For the rest of us, put the curler on your top lashes and press. Hold for a quick count of fifteen, pressing the curler several times while you are counting. Do this on one eye, put on your mascara, then curl the other eye. After you put on one coat on the upper lashes of each eye, let that coat dry. Go on to the next step in your routine, then return and put on another coat. It is very important to let the coats of mascara dry between applications. This will prevent mascara buildup that will make your lashes bunch. I sometimes like to put translucent powder on my lashes in between applications of mascara. It seems to make the mascara hold better and last longer.

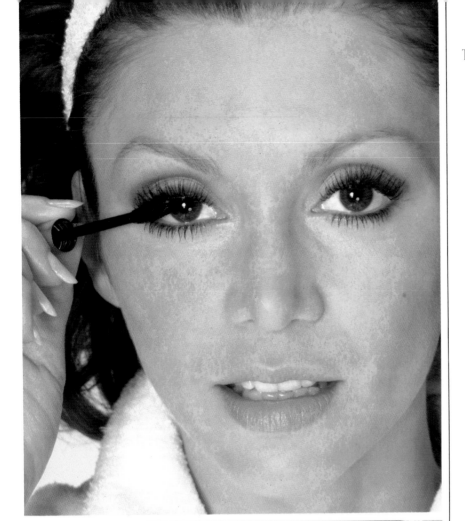

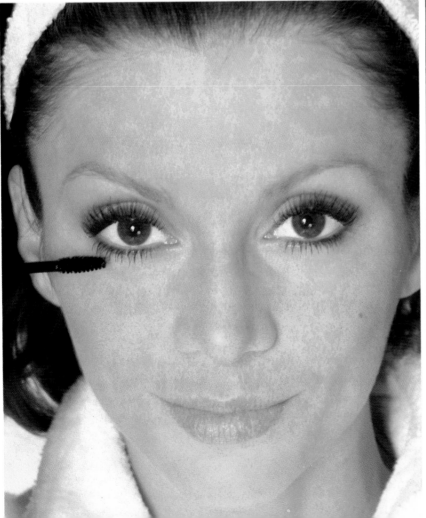

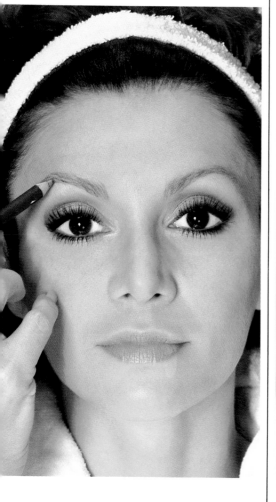

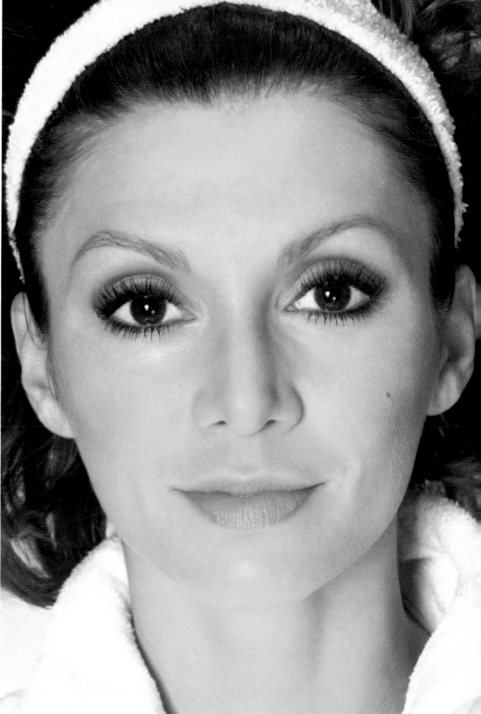

9

9. On most days I do not bother with using an eyebrow pencil. But if you have gaps in your eyebrows, take your pencil and with light, feathery strokes fill in your eyebrows. Use a pencil the same color as your brows (don't try to change the color with a pencil—that is best done by dyeing eyebrows, which we will talk about later) and make tiny, featherlike lines, much like the hairs in your brows. Never draw a single line: It looks silly and just like what it is—a line drawn through your eyebrows. Lightly and subtly feather in the hairs that would have been there had your eyebrows been perfect. And while you are doing this, remember that the light touch is important.

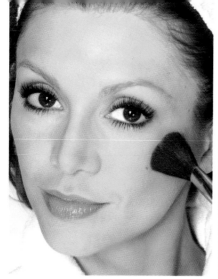

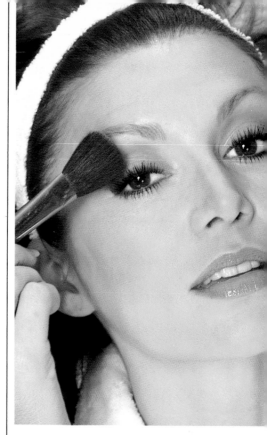

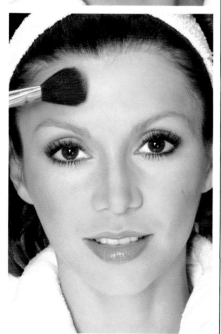

10. If you want, you may now brush some powder blush and translucent powder all over your face to further set your makeup.

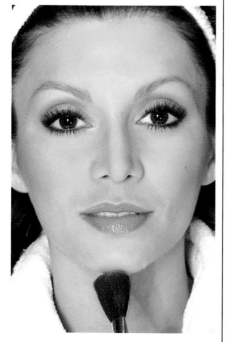

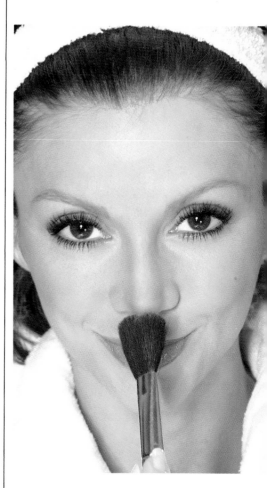

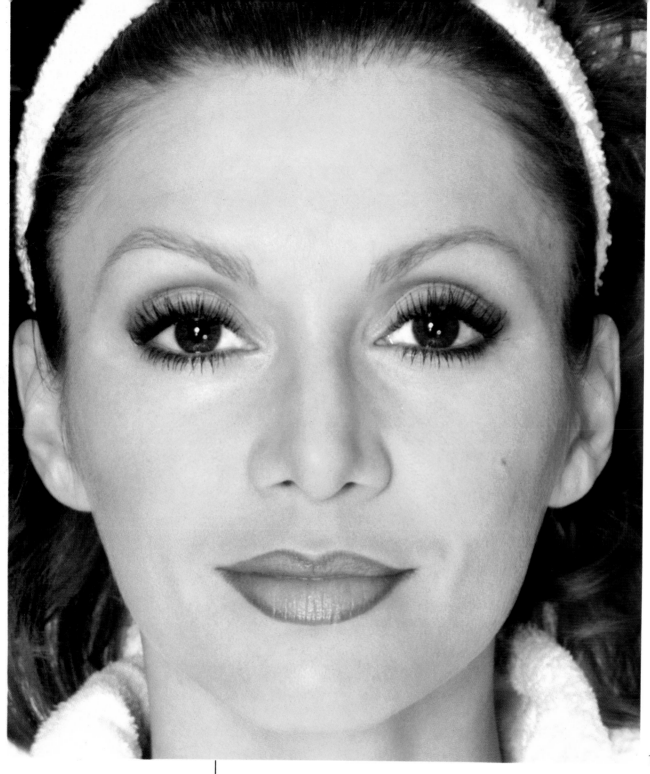

11. Lip time. To make sure my lips are clean, I blot them on a tissue. Don't wet your lips before applying lipstick—it will inhibit smooth coverage. I line my lips with a lip liner pencil a shade darker than my glossy lipstick (not above my lips but on them). I then smudge the line with my fingertips or a cotton swab to soften the outline, and fill in with my wand lipstick. Sometimes I put a dot of light foundation in the middle of my lower lip to give it an extra glow.

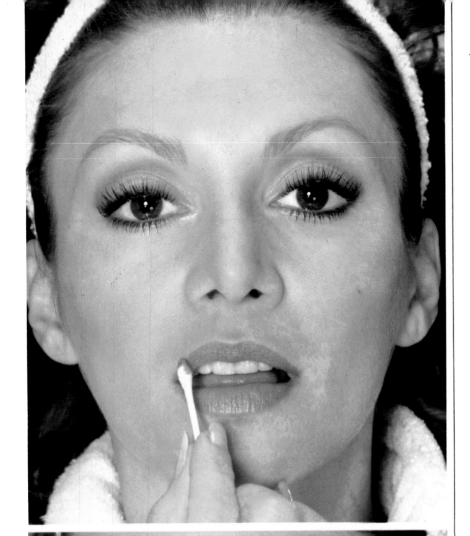

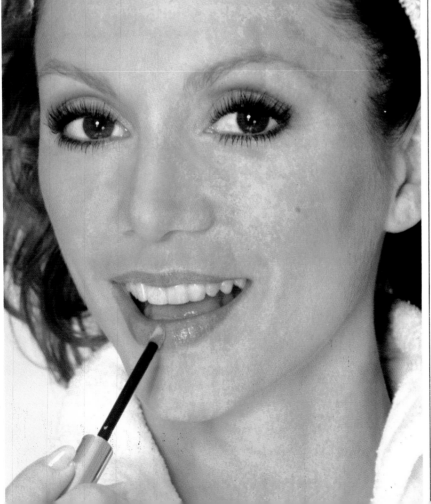

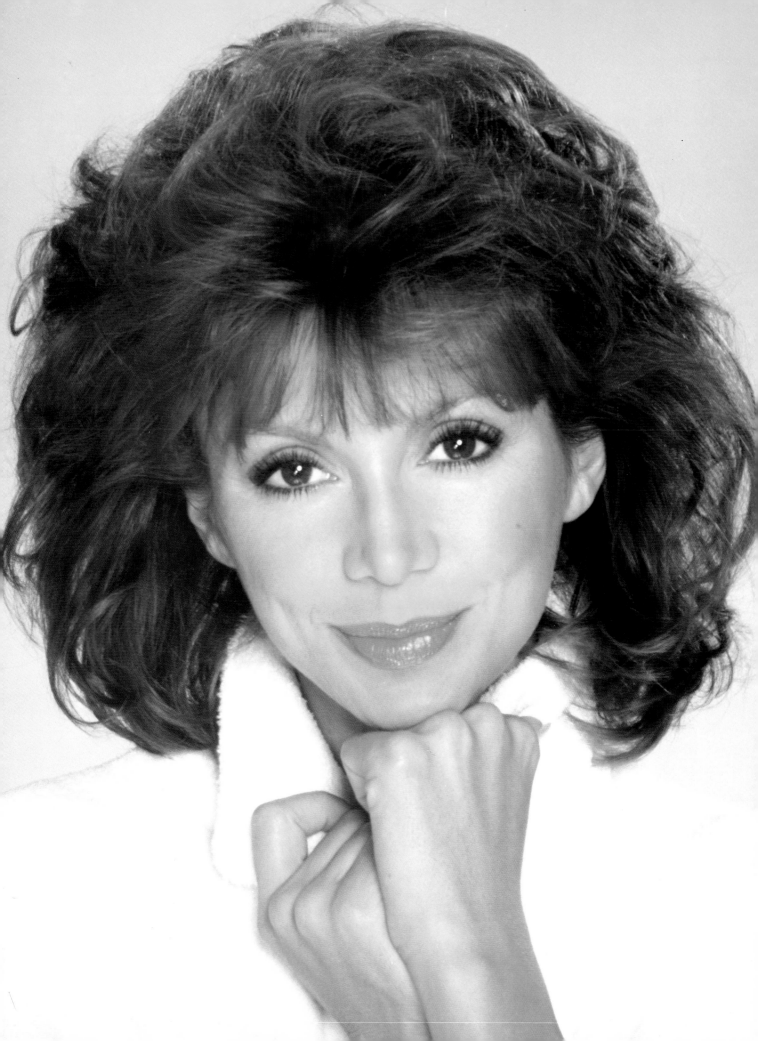

Was I right? This took, at the most, ten minutes. Don't groan in disbelief—be patient. With some practice, you'll have it down in no time.

Now take a little test. Look in the mirror. If you can't see your skin through your foundation, you have too much of it on your face. If you can see lines between your different creams (highlighter, concealer, foundation, blush) you need more practice in blending. If you can see the brush strokes of your blush or your eye shadow, you put too much on. Next time, start out by putting less of everything on your face.

And remember, the "painting a canvas" analogy still holds— put on your makeup in layers. You *layer* the foundation, you *layer* the shadows, you *layer* the blush, a little at a time.

One more thing: These steps are not rules carved in stone—they are guidelines and suggestions that should work for everyone. But if you need to change a step or leave one out—do it! The beauty of this routine is not only its effectiveness but also its flexibility.

Finished ten-minute makeup

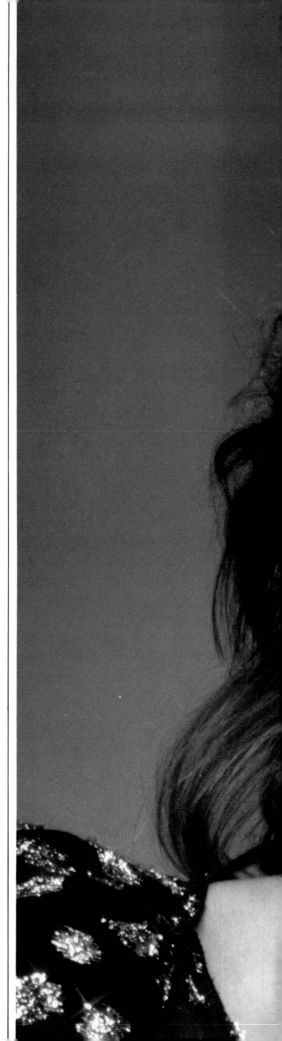

The Fresh Nighttime Face

There are times when you will want a more glamorous makeup than the ten-minute makeup routine. Regardless of the shape of your eyes, nose, lips or face, with a little time and understanding you can achieve your own great nighttime face (see page 113).

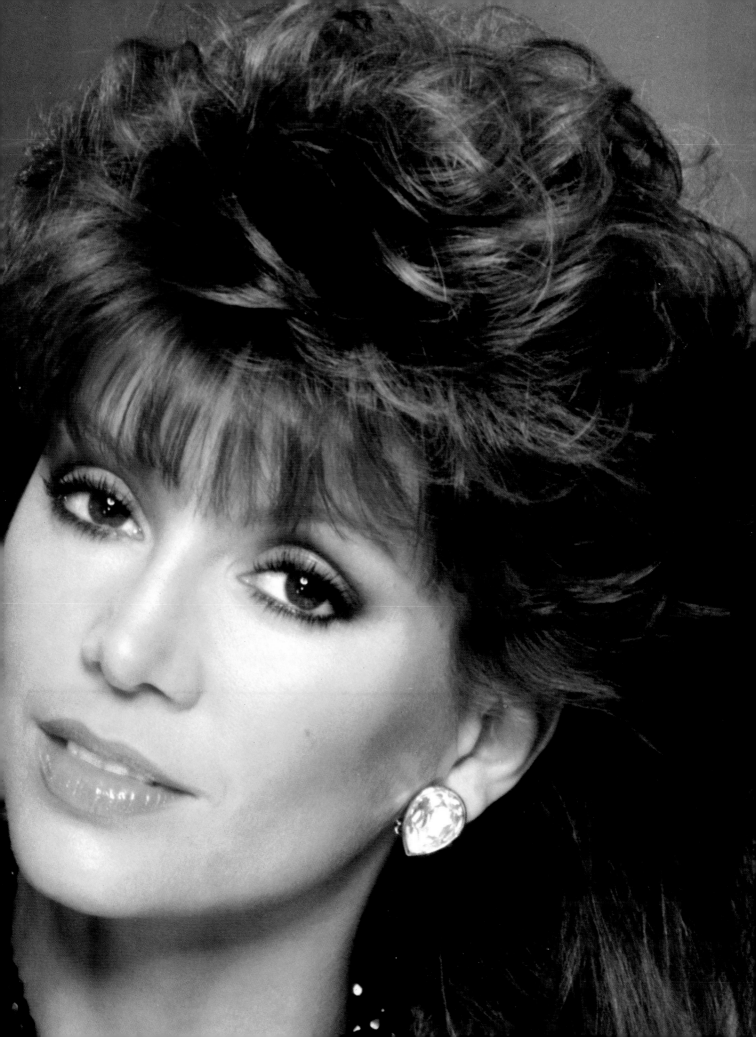

TYPES OF COMPLEXIONS AND FEATURES

In order to put on your makeup in a way that best suits your face, you need to know not only what makeup is and how to apply it, but also what kind of complexion and what shape features you have.

Skin Types and Makeup

1. If you have skin that is basically oily—use a liquid, water-based foundation.

2. If you have skin that is basically dry—use an oil-based liquid or cream foundation.

3. If you have problem skin—you need a nongreasy foundation, since this type of skin is usually very oily. Medicated foundations can be helpful.

That said, remember that since most women have combination skin, the best foundation for us is a water-based foundation in a color close to that of your own skin. So before you diagnose yourself as having dry or oily skin, take stock. Use the preceding guidelines only if your skin exhibits true and definite characteristics of the various skin types.

Skin Tones and Makeup

• *Ruddy:* Use a foundation with beige or green, no pink or rose.

• *Sallow:* Use a foundation with peach or pink; you may also want to use an under-foundation primer to even out the tones in your skin.

• *Olive:* Use a tawny foundation.

• *Oriental:* Use a foundation with pink in it.

• *Black:* Use a foundation with orange in it.

IF YOU HAVE A RUDDY COMPLEXION

The best way to describe this kind of skin is skin that always seems to be excited; it's a pink blush but it can also be a little splotchy. The ruddiness usually appears at the tip of the nose, the chin, the cheeks and the forehead. What you need to remember about this type of skin is that you want to even out the color, but you don't want to lose that wonderful glow—just subdue it a bit. So use a soft beige foundation with a touch of green in it (I don't mean a touch of green food coloring but an essence of green that compliments the other colors in your skin). You can also use the under-foundation primer that is made to even out the tones in your skin. Above all, be proud of this look—it is a friendly, radiating glow that needs only to be evened out, not erased.

IF YOU HAVE A SALLOW COMPLEXION

Sallow is a skin tone with a yellow cast to it. What you may want to do is add some color to it, but you don't want to create a color for your face that is different from your body. So the foundation used for sallow skin must be subtle, yet effective. Use a cream with a touch of peach or a light touch of pink. I use one with pink and tawny in it; it blends with my coloring but also gives me a little touch of sunshine (that's from the tawny). I always buy my foundation in tawny beige.

IF YOU HAVE AN OLIVE COMPLEXION

This is a combination sallow and tan-looking skin. All you need to do is use a foundation that matches your skin with a touch of rose in it.

IF YOU HAVE ORIENTAL SKIN

Oriental skin is usually sallow with strong yellow tones. A foundation with pink in it is most flattering.

IF YOU HAVE BLACK SKIN

Foundation for black skin should have some orange or red in it to give the skin a healthy glow. There are now several lines of cosmetics for black skin that contain these complimentary colors (check with your local department store). Generally black skin is attractive with many of the same colors as yellow or brown skin. And the principles are the same—be subtle, blend, moisturize, and develop a routine that best accentuates your features and minimizes your faults.

IF YOU HAVE MATURE SKIN

The most common mistake mature women make is to put on more makeup, figuring that heavier coverage will make them look better. Wrong! Older skin needs much more moisturizing plus a creamy emulsion—makeup that has more body to it and more pigment, with opaque but not masklike coverage. The worst sight is an attractive, older woman with so much makeup on that she accentuates the lines and the other aging characteristics of her skin—however minimal they may be. In this case, less is definitely more. You don't want to put on your regular makeup in a thicker manner, because all you will get is an increased definition of the lines on your face. Wear a makeup that has more body to it, one that you will use in the same amount as you always did, but one that will now give you the added coverage you need.

Face Shapes

There is a lot of talk in magazines and among makeup artists about "fixing" faces with makeup, sort of a "corrective" philosophy which holds that no matter what shape your face is, you can make it look different, somehow better, making it adhere to whatever is "in style" or "in vogue" this year. This sort of "Don't worry, we can make your face look just like Helen of Troy's" philosophy makes me crazy.

No matter what shape your face is, you can make *it* look beautiful by accentuating your best features and minimizing those you don't love as much.

IF YOU HAVE A ROUND FACE

If you want to minimize some of your face's roundness (but not to try to create a different shape), learn to use your contour just at the edges of your face, from your jawline and out about a quarter of an inch or so. Then blend the cream into your foundation so there is no line between them. Be aware that this is not such an easy maneuver, and you could end up looking like a round-faced lady with dirt around her face. It's happened to me—so just practice until you feel you have it right.

For blush on your round face, take your powder blush and brush two parenthesis-shaped strokes on either side of your face, and one on your chin.

ROUND FACE

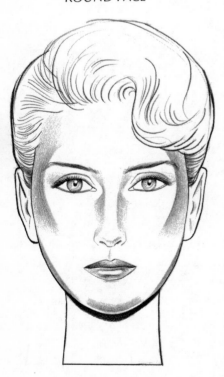

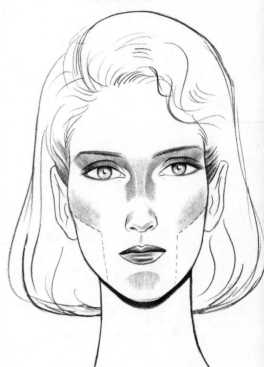

LONG FACE

IF YOU HAVE A LONG FACE

If you want to widen a long face a bit, put lighter foundation on your cheeks and out to the jawline. Now blend. Then take your blush and brush some on the top (not tip) of your nose, under your eyebrows and on your chin. This should give your face the illusion of added width in the center.

IF YOU HAVE A TRIANGULAR FACE

(I have to tell you that I am always wary of people who use this description, because your face really is not a triangle—it is merely shaped narrower at the top and wider at the bottom; but for lack of a better term, I use this one.) To minimize a triangular face, shadow the sides of your face from the cheekbones down with your contour, then blend. Put some light foundation at the top of both sides of your forehead and blend again.

Now brush your blush in a parenthesis around the side of each your eyes—create a brush stroke that goes from the top of your eyebrow across your cheekbone, ending before the nose.

TRIANGULAR FACE

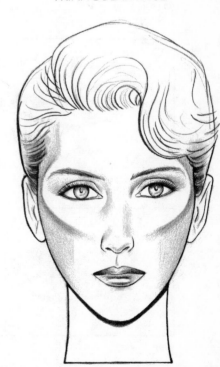

Eyes

Making up my eyes is my favorite part of the makeup routine because it seems to give a focus to my entire look. The eyes are a lot of fun—they are where I "play," where I like to try new things and am always in awe of what a difference the most subtle of makeups can make. And if it is true that your eyes are the mirror of your soul, then you want your soul to look as wonderful as possible.

Just as you did with foundation, it is important to discover your *basic eye look*. This look should not try to alter the shape of your eyes, it should only enhance them. Stick with what you have. The point is to make your own shape look as pretty as possible.

I believe that the eyes are what one notices first about a person, so I always keep this in mind when I make them up. But I don't want them to stand out so much that no one will notice anything else about me. Nor do I want them to resemble garage doors (more about those later); I simply want my eyes to be beautiful.

THE BASIC EYE

This is the makeup you will probably wear on your eyes 95 percent of the time. It can carry you from morning to night, although there

SMALL EYES

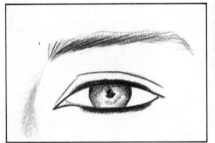

STEP 1.

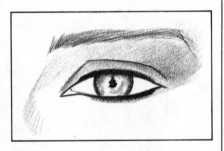

STEP 2.

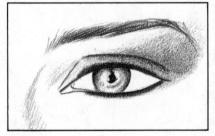

STEP 3.

are options I will discuss later for making up your eyes for particular occasions. The basic eye, which is described in the Ten-Minute Makeup Routine (page 81) will work for your easy, daytime look no matter what shape your eyes are, because it is such a minimal yet attractive and effective look. When we discuss other tricks for eye makeup, there will be differences of technique and application depending on the shape of your eyes.

Do remember a couple of things. Apply *undereye concealer* (again, see the Ten-Minute Makeup Routine—page 81) right after you have moisturized your face but before you put on your foundation. And for constant shadows under the eyes, try to get more sleep. Doctors say that the vast majority of the circles people develop under their eyes are from lack of sleep. If your circles are a result of a sinus problem or other medical condition, don't just conceal and ignore them. See a doctor.

For *undereye puffiness,* use a highlighter or your light foundation underneath your eyes to refract light and make it look as if your "undereye" area is even with your face; again, an optical illusion.

Some women like to dye their eyelashes so they don't have to wear mascara much of the time. It is usually a safe procedure, especially with the vegetable dyes now on the market. But please let a professional do it. You don't want to take a chance on damaging your eyes.

SMALL EYES

Most women who have small eyes want to make them appear larger. Many makeup artists feel that lining small eyes makes them look narrower. I don't agree. I like to see narrow eyes lined—I think it punches them out (to coin a phrase), makes the white look whiter and makes them more evident. But there is a difference in lining small eyes, and that is to make the line soft, sort of smudged (use a soft eye pencil). So:

1. Line your eyes with a soft creamy eye pencil. Don't let the bottom and top lines touch in the corner of each eye; stop just before.

2. Then use a dark shadow on your lid, extending all the way to your brow bone. Blend it with your fingertips.

3. Put your highlighter (or your lightest foundation) between

your brows and the edge of the shadow. Blend that in—see how large your eyes look.

4. If your small eyes are also close together, try putting a touch of light foundation at both corners to make them look farther apart.

HOODED EYES
(SOMETIMES CALLED DROOPING-LID EYES)

1. Add to the basic eye by putting eye shadow on the entire lid, continuing it a little beyond the crease above your eye.

2. Now put a lighter shade or a highlighter under your eyebrow. Make sure your eyes are outlined in a dark pencil. These steps will work for you no matter what shape your eyes are.

To compensate for one drooping lid, you need to accentuate that eye more than the other but in a subtle way. Let me explain. The idea is not to overemphasize the better eye so that no one will notice that your other lid droops a bit; the idea is to make up the drooping eye just a bit more than the better eye so that they will look even. So, on the eyelid that droops:

1. Use your light foundation on the top drooping lid and make a dark line with your eye pencil in the crease above your eye. Smudge with a cotton swab.

2. Now take your eye pencil and make a wider than usual line above the lashes and under the eye to enlarge your eye. Now you have taken attention away from the droop but not from the eye itself.

HOODED EYES

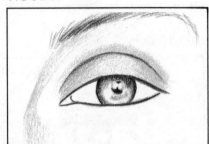

STEP 1.

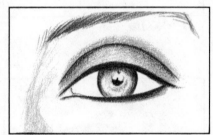

STEP 2.

ONE DROOPING LID

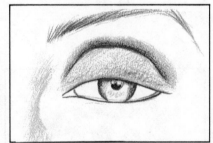

STEP 1.

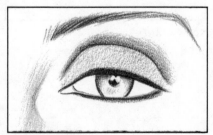

STEP 2.

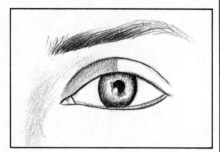

STEP 1.

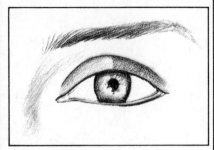

STEP 2.

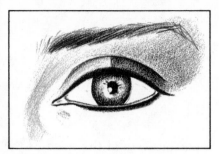

STEPS 3. AND 4.

LARGE EYES

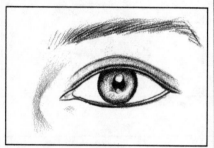

STEPS 1. AND 2.

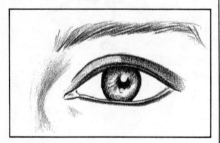

STEP 3.

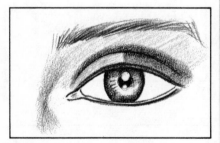

STEPS 4. AND 5.

DEEP-SET EYES

Take your basic eye makeup and do the following:

1. Always take your light foundation or a light-colored beige or pink eye shadow and spread it on your eyelid from the inside corner of your eye to the middle of the lid (half the eye will then be covered in this color).

2. Now use a darker shade (which can be the same shade as you may want to use under your eyebrow, or just a darker shade of your beige) on the other half of your lid (the outer half, from the middle to the outside of your eye).

3. Always outline your eyes, top and bottom eyelids, with a creamy eye-lining pencil.

4. Brush a dash of your blush along your brow bone.

LARGE EYES

Everybody should have your problem. This is every woman's dream —to have large eyes. Making up these eyes is easy, and the results are beautiful. Take your basic eye and:

1. Add another line above your eyelid with a soft pencil in a dark shade (assuming you have your penciled-in mascara line).

2. Take your basic eye and add eye shadow over the entire lid.

3. Take your darker shade of shadow and cover the lid from the middle of the eye to the outside.

4. Brush the darker shadow in the crease above the eye.

5. Brush a light shadow or your blush under your brow.

ALMOND-SHAPED EYES

Mine! As I told you before, I used to try to make them round, but try as I did, they were always almond, especially when I took off my eye makeup. I finally realized that this shape is perfectly fine, so I just follow my basic eye. Sometimes I accentuate my eyes, but I'm getting ahead of myself. I'll explain all that when we get to the fun eyes.

ORIENTAL EYES

Take the basic eye and add your lightest foundation just under the brow line, or, if you prefer, leave a space between the brow and one-quarter inch below it to give the area above the eye added height. Now take your lightest eye shadow and brush your eyelid from the inner corner of the eye to the middle of the eyelid. Take a darker shade of the same color and brush it on what's left of your eyelid. When using a liner, make sure the lines don't meet or your eyes will look smaller than they are. Take the line from the outside of the eye to the middle, both on the lid and the undereye.

ROUND EYES

Eyes are supposed to be round. If you have such eyes, use the basic eye makeup, and have a nice day.

THE KNOCKOUT EYE

That's not a black eye you got in a fight. It's that fabulous, sparkly, glamorous eye that you want to wear only for a "knockout" affair—please, never to the supermarket or the bookstore—they'll never understand. And why should they? The knockout eye is appropriate any evening you dress with a sense of drama. It should complement your wardrobe and your environment. But remember, don't go crazy. Amplify your eye, but don't lose your basic eye makeup that accentuates and enhances your face. Use some discretion as to when to stop, or you'll look as if someone did knock you out. Here's how to do it:

1. Take your basic daytime eye, and reapply everything you did that morning except the mascara/liner in your lashes.

2. Take your basic dark pencil and line the very inside corner of your eye (you are drawing a little "v"), and then extend this emphasis upward in a darker shade of shadow. Here you can add an eye shadow that has a little more color in it—a deep purple, a deep rose or a taupe.

3. Add another coat or two (remembering to wait between applications) of your mascara.

4. If you like iridescent shades of eye shadow, or you want to try a colored mascara, this is the time to do it. But go easy—you

THE KNOCKOUT EYE

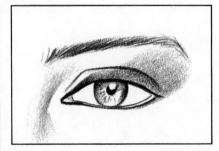

STEP 2.

don't want to end up looking too trendy or comical. There is a fine line between breathtaking and foolish. Don't cross it. The effect to aim for is one of glamour that also brings out the best in your eyes.

Eyes You Never Want to Have

GARAGE DOOR EYES
Whenever I see eyes painted with one color (blue-black lids) and I watch them open and close, I can't help but think of garage doors. Don't do it. Be subtle—if you must use a color, use it gently and blend it in.

OWL EYES
You've seen them—white lids, white undereye concealer, white pencil—the works. It may have worked in the fifties, but it is outdated and not flattering. Leave white for the walls.

BLACK EYES
This is not the "knockout" eye, nor is it a "knocked-out eye." It's when the lid is covered in black shadow, the eyes outlined in black pencil and black eye liner, and the mascara thickly layered. It's too much. A little black inside the eye or on your lashes is fine; and if you have a dark complexion and dark hair, outline your eyes in black.

TECHNICOLOR EYES
Blue eyelids, green eye liner, orange shadow on the brows, three colors above the eyelid—again it's overdone. The best eye makeup is subtle, when the application is hardly noticeable.

Eyebrows

I am sure you have heard this before—consider your eyebrows the frame for your eyes. It's true. Look at it this way: If your eyes are a beautiful, mesmerizing picture, you certainly don't want to overwhelm them with the frame. As in a good piece of art, the frame is a compliment to the work. If you like your eyebrows full, natural, and you don't like to tweeze them, don't. Leave them as they are. If they are very bushy and tend to be unruly (but you still don't want to tweeze them), take an eyebrow brush, brush them well, then spray the brush with hair spray and apply to your brows. This will help make them more manageable.

But you should be aware that as a woman grows older, as many parts of her body will begin to move down, her eyebrows are also going to look heavy and low. As we age, our faces begin to sag a bit, and sagging eyebrows really take away from sparkling, full and bright eyes. So for mature women who have always preferred not to shape the eyebrows, reform. Just try to pluck them at the bottom of the brow to clean and lift them up a bit.

I always suggest that you go to a professional just once to get your eyebrows shaped properly. She can make sure that your brows frame your eyes as they should, in a flattering and attractive way, and can see that both brows are the same shape (I have a hard time making the shapes match myself). Then you can maintain this shape by periodically cleaning the hairs that grow in.

For those of you who do want to shape your brows, there are ways in which your eyebrows cannot only frame but actually enhance your eyes and minimize their drawbacks. For example, if your eyes seem to slant down, sort of "sadly," you can minimize the slope by shaping your eyebrows into straighter lines (the effect is much like a puppeteer who can pick up a puppet on one side and lift it a little). If you have evenly set eyes, start your brow where your eye starts and end it where your eye ends. If you have eyes that are widely set, start your eyebrow closer to your nose and end it where your eye ends. This will seem to bring your eyes closer together. For eyes that are set closely together, start your eyebrow a little bit after your eye, to make your eyes look farther apart.

TWEEZING

Again, the good thing about going to a professional for a tweezing is that she can shape your eyebrows to flatter and compliment your eyes. From then on, when you pick up tweezers, all you have to do is follow the pattern she has set (you may find that after a few weeks you will want another professional tweeze, but you really can keep it up by yourself).

Remember—tweezers just sit around in makeup drawers and pick up a lot of dust and dirt. So be sure to always dip your tweezers in astringent or in alcohol before using them.

When you are ready to tweeze your eyebrows, put some astringent on a cotton ball (again alcohol will do as well, even better) and wipe your eyebrows with it. Now start tweezing in the direction in which the hairs grow. As you tweeze try to follow the line that is there—merely clean out the hairs that have grown in. Stop every so often and see how you have done. Sometimes it is better to stop and wait until the next day to continue. First, this process can hurt and irritate your skin and make your eyes tear, so stopping may appeal to you. Second, it is better to leave some extra hairs than to tweeze too many and have to wait for them to grow back in.

A word about *electrolysis*. I think it is fine for facial hair that is unsightly and bothersome to you. But I believe that eyebrows should be tweezed. Electrolysis is a permanent solution and you may want to leave yourself the option of changing the shape of your eyebrows.

Another method that some people like is to remove eyebrow hair by waxing. But I think this process should be done by a professional. It's safer that way. I have talked to too many women who have burned their skin with hot wax. So leave that to the pros and shape your eyebrows at home by tweezing.

COLORING YOUR EYEBROWS

If you feel you need to color your eyebrows because they do not suit the color of your hair or your complexion, it is relatively easy to do at home. I use a facial cream hair lightener, which I think is the cheapest, safest and easiest way to lighten your eyebrows.

Mix the lightener according to the directions on the box. Stand in front of a mirror, apply the cream gently to your brows and watch it. The color will change from black to brown to red to blond. Wipe it off at the stage you want, before it reaches the color of your hair, because eyebrows should be a shade darker, otherwise the whole world will know you have been coloring them! Remember, coloring does dry out your brows, so don't do it too often. And when you take off the lightener, apply moisturizer to your eyebrows and leave it there. I always put moisturizer on my eyebrows just as I do on my face at night. It is a good way to avoid dry, flaky skin in that area.

A word about disciplining your eyebrows. I really believe it can be done. I didn't start tweezing my brows until my late teens when I was modeling. But I did, on my mother's advice, start brushing them when I was twelve—every now and then with my own tiny brush. I thought it was such a special thing to do. And I believe it helped make them as pretty and easy to maintain as they are today.

Lips

After you have applied your foundation, your contour (if you choose to use it) and/or your highlighter, and after you have done your eyes, it's time to work on your lips. Some lip tips follow.

How much you do with your lips is completely up to you. There is no wrong or right answer as to whether to wear lipstick—only wrong and right ways to apply it. It's up to you how you want to treat your lips. But whatever you decide, here are some tricks of the trade to show your lips to their best advantage.

An important thing to think about concerning your lips is that there are two extremes, neither one of which, as is often the case, is terrific. One is the naked lip. I really believe that after the age of sixteen, every woman needs a little color on her lips, even if it is only a sheer gloss with a touch of pink in it. First of all, everyone needs something that moisturizes the lips. Secondly, the extra shine that lipstick (or gloss, or petroleum jelly, which, by the way, is a terrific moisturizer—it gives your lips a wonderful glow) provides is a touch that your face should not be without.

A face without something on the lips really looks undone, unfinished—as if you forgot something. This is particularly so for women whose makeup routine is the simplest one—a little mascara and blush on good clean skin—because naked lips will make the whole face seem wan, while a little gloss can pick up the entire look.

The other extreme is a lip that is overdone, that screams for attention and gets it, at the expense of your face. You really don't want your lips to precede you into a room, do you? Yet many women so overline and overcolor their lips that their mouth is the first (and sometimes the only) thing you notice about their whole appearance.

Another mistake some women make is to choose lipstick without any consideration for their foundation and their blush. This is not a good idea because the lipstick can then clash with the rest of your makeup. And even if the difference is subtle, believe me, it will still be noticeable. So if you use a tawny blush, choose a lipstick from tawny to bronze to beige to compliment your makeup. If you use a rose foundation and a rose blush, you need to use a lipstick within the range of rose to pink that corresponds with your foundation.

Yet another misconception about lipstick is that it should match the clothes you wear. This is simply not true, and can in fact make you look rather silly. First of all, the days of matching everything are gone. Fashion has for many years advised that the natural, more casual look (rather than the detailed, precise, everything-dyed-the-same-color look) is the right one for everyone. You can choose to wear what you want to wear—you need not have to make sure that everything you own, whether it be clothes or makeup, be the same color. Shades and textures that compliment one another—yes. But gone are the days when your shoes, gloves, hat, purse, dress, lipstick and nail polish all had to match.

You don't have to—and shouldn't, really—change your lip color every time you change your clothes. You don't do it with your hair or with your foundation, so why with your lipstick? Unless it is a special occasion (usually an evening gala where unusual shades of color might be appropriate), stick to the lipstick that compliments your face. The lesson here is also this: If you find a foundation and blush color that go with your complexion and hair, and you find a lipstick that compliments these colors, chances are that all these colors will go with almost everything you wear.

PUTTING ON LIPSTICK

If you have the perfect mouth, then you have the option of following your own lip line and not using a pencil to line your lips. Merely brush the lipstick (either with a lipstick brush if you are using a tube lipstick, or with a wand) on your lips.

Even though I always use a lip pencil because I think it is so attractive to clearly define the lip line, I use it to do just that—define the *existing* line of *my* lips. I do not redraw my lip line. I really believe that if you have a certain lip shape, it is going to be self-defeating to try to draw an exceedingly different shape on your lips. In other words, think about trying to create a new mouth—and then drinking a sip of tea. Chances are you'll soon be left with half a new mouth and half an old one! And what about kissing someone, and finding your new mouth on his lips and your old one on yours! Getting the point? Why not stick with your own and make the most of it, rather than attempting to draw a different lip shape that will be obviously made up and look unnatural.

CONTOURING LIPS

I do believe, however, that you can do certain things to create more of a visual balance to your lips, without having to create a new mouth. For example, if you have a small upper lip (or two small lips), you can take a lipstick pencil or a lipstick brush with a color slightly darker than the one you use on the rest of your lips, and slightly (minutely, really) go above your lip line, sticking close to the edge. If you decide to go this route, make sure you have put foundation and powder over your lip line (this will make the lip line smooth and will not define it as separate from the foundation).

Now put your everyday lipstick (or gloss—in which case your lip pencil can be a medium rose or a peach or a brown) on the rest of your lips.

A good test is if you can see the lip line from any distance at all, it isn't working.

If you want your upper lip to look more protruding (I love this look—it makes the lips very sensual, very sexy) do this with your highlighter: Notice the cleft, or indentation, between your nose and upper lip. Put a lighter foundation or a highlighter there—it reflects light and makes the upper lip look as if it is protruding.

FACES YOU MAY NEED

Do you remember the basic Ten-Minute Makeup Routine? That is how I start out every day. Thus, you'll never catch me leaving my house at nine in the morning with my nighttime face on—I'd look ridiculous! And it is unnecessary—that's what touch-ups are for.

The following are tricks and hints for touching up at lunchtime and in the evening, and the secrets of creating a fresh nighttime face.

Touch-up Tricks

Over the years I have learned many "tricks of the trade" for quick pick-me-ups in makeup. Often when I find myself shooting a film, by the middle of the day my makeup is disappearing, my face seems to have lost its sparkle, and I find it is time for a makeup pick-me-up.

The same thing has happened to me in my private life. I return home from a day of work on the set at MGM (where we film "Dallas"), and I find that I have to be at a dinner in ten minutes, or I have to do an interview in five. Under these circumstances there is no chance to do my makeup over, yet my face feels and looks wan, tired, somehow just not right.

At these times, I have found several things I can do to quickly and easily make the best of a tired situation. I have picked up these tricks from many sources—from fellow actors, from my many makeup artists over the years, from my photographers and from my girlfriends. So here are some tips that may come in handy.

LUNCHTIME TOUCH-UP

Sometimes when I am having lunch in a restaurant and go to the ladies' room, I look in the mirror and find that my face looks exhausted. Rather than panic, I take out my makeup bag (see page 123) —after years of experience, I have come up with a bag I carry absolutely everywhere, and it has never let me down. Thus, within reach of the bag and its contents, I touch up my face. These are the steps:

1. First I take out my saline solution and put a drop in each eye. Immediately the redness disappears and my eyes open up as if I had just woken up from a nap.

2. Now I take out my tiny sample bottle of astringent, put some on a tissue and pat down my forehead, the center of my nose and the side of both nostrils, because these spots have by this time gotten somewhat oily and need attention. These simple strokes, followed by a touch of pressed powder from my compact, somehow make my whole face look renewed and clean.

3. I take out my lightest foundation (you can take out any foundation you have on hand), and put a dot on the center of each eyelid and blend it in. This immediately opens up my eyes. If I feel I need more foundation (just a touch—not a complete reapplication which may give me a masklike look), I take my small bottle of skin-tone foundation and touch up the spots that need it with my fingertips, and powder over those areas.

4. Next I look at my eyes, and if I was wearing some eye shadow when I left the house in the morning, I touch up a little on the eyelid for extra coverage. The eye shadow I carry in my makeup bag is a light shade, because this lighter color opens up my eyes. If you like the look, add another stroke of the brush with a darker shadow in the crease above the eye.
Now I take out my kohl pencil to reapply the liner on the very inside corner of my eyes. This, too, will instantly perk up the eyes—they will look reborn.

5. Time for the blusher. Use your retractable brush and add some light strokes over the cheekbones, above your eyes (just under the brows), on the tip of your nose, your chin, and on your neck. It will give you an overall healthy glow.

6. Check your mascara—if it is caking, try to separate the lashes with the eyelash brush in your bag. Otherwise, you can simply add yet another layer of mascara.

7. Lips need a quick touch-up as well, especially if you have just eaten. (Some women aren't used to touching up their makeup at lunchtime but are in the habit of reapplying their lipstick at the table. Don't do it. I have always felt that putting on lipstick at the table is impolite and unattractive. So if you are going to apply lipstick, excuse yourself to a restroom and do it there.)

The first thing to do is to clean the lips by blotting them with a napkin or a tissue. Next I lightly coat them with vitamin E stick for some nourishment. Then, if I have used a lip liner, I reapply that line with my pencil and blend it with my fingertip so that the color looks continuous. Then I put clear gloss on my lips. If you only have petroleum jelly, that will do just fine; I have met many actresses who only use petroleum jelly on their lips because it keeps them soft and looks as shiny as lipstick.

Sometimes I also put a dot of my light foundation on the center of my lower lip for added sparkle.

That's it. This whole process doesn't take five minutes—I am often out of there and back at the table before anyone realizes I left.

THE NIGHTTIME FACE TOUCH-UP
(WORKING FROM THE DAYTIME FACE)

For evening, if you don't have the time to start all over again, you must work with the daytime face you made up earlier. Don't worry about overdoing your face and damaging that skin you have so carefully nourished. First of all, the cosmetics you are using on your face should not be harming your skin, especially if you remove them each and every night before you go to bed. Second, the amount of cosmetics you are using is really minimal—light foundation, minimal color coverage, light touches everywhere, so your skin should be fine underneath. Third, even if you have touched up your face at lunchtime, you did so gently and lightly, and by now your skin will have absorbed some of the makeup.

Nighttime is drama time. No matter what you are doing, your face can be made up in a more dramatic and obvious way than in the daytime. That does not mean you will look like a clown. It merely means that because nighttime light is dimmer and usually electric, very different from the brightness and harshness of sunlight, you can get away with more emphatic makeup. Remember, there is nothing wrong with wanting to stand out in a crowd; in fact, making up for nighttime accomplishes this very thing.

The most important change from the daytime face to the nighttime face is the way I treat my eyes. Emphasizing the eyes is an easy and very effective way to punch up your nighttime makeup. Here goes:

1. First I reapply the pencil line over the lashes (not the pencil-in-mascara line that was made between and in the lashes, but the one made with the soft eye pencil above the lashes).

2. Now I reapply my darker shade of eye shadow, sweeping it from the crease of the eye up to the brow (leaving the section directly on the eyelid covered with the lighter eye shadow).

3. Now I probably need to apply a lighter powder under each eye because the day's fatigue is taking its toll under my eyes (sometimes I use my concealer wand, and then powder over it). You can also powder there with blush.

4. Optional—You can use your darker foundation (or contour cream) just at the top of and below your cheekbones (this is recommended only for those of you who have learned how to contour and feel comfortable using this technique).

5. Now I use my powder blush. Remember, I started out my day with a cream blush with a touch of powder blush and translucent powder over it. I now use only the powder blush, because trying to put cream blush over my powder will result in a mess. Besides, at this time of the day, with the receding light, I can afford to use the powder blush, and use it with a slightly heavier hand than in the morning. I put powder blush at the tip of my chin, at the tip of my nose, and a touch under my eyebrows for an added healthy glow, and a guaranteed dramatic impact I adore.

6. I end this short routine with a touch of my water-filled atomizer to set my just-touched-up nighttime face.

THE COCKTAIL EYE

This is the basic eye that needs a pick-me-up at five or six o'clock. It is particularly important for the working woman who leaves work but has no time to go home and redo her makeup before a cocktail meeting or dinner date. It is easy to create because the foundation eye makeup is already on your eye. Take your beige eye shadow and cover your whole lid. Add a darker shade in the crease of your eye, and a highlighter or a blusher under the brow. You can also, if you choose, brush a light pink or a very light beige shadow in the inside corner of your lid. Redo your eye pencil (not the one with the mascara on it in your lashes—that one stays all day and night). Then add another coat of mascara.

THE FRESH NIGHTTIME FACE

When you have the luxury of starting your nighttime face from scratch, you can have a face that is truly different from your daytime look. You now have the chance to create the mood you want for this particular evening. And this takes some deliberate thought.

I have always tried to make sure that my evening makeup, my evening face, corresponds to what I am wearing, where I am going, how I am feeling, and the image I want to present that night. This is very different from the daytime face. During the day I use my most simple and attractive makeup, but I can take more liberties with my nighttime face. This is the time for fantasy, for daring. But, as with everything, there is a time and place for this "different," accentuated and not-that-subtle face. An evening gown with elaborate, dramatic makeup may not be appropriate for a sit-down dinner in someone's home, unless such an elegant black-tie atmosphere was specifically planned by the host and hostess. Again, if you are going where people are more conservative in life style, it does not mean you have to pretend to be someone you are not. But you don't have to make a point of being different. I feel that it is fine to stand out in a room, to call attention to yourself. But this attention has to be in line with the mood of the evening—it must, above all, be appropriate.

So if you know where you are going, if you know what to expect, be sure that your dress and makeup are suitable for the occasion. This merely means giving your makeup as much thought as you give the gown or dress or suit you will wear.

And the options are many. If you are going to a dressy affair, you can dress up your nighttime face with intense eye shadows, with iridescent cheek powders, and with darker lipstick that makes your mouth stand out. But you may want to do just the opposite—tone down your face to create a delicate evening makeup that gives you a more fragile look. Nighttime may be the time to use your makeup to play a little with reality. (For finished Fresh Nighttime Face, see page 95.)

TIPS FOR SPECIAL PROBLEMS

Skin Shine

There are some skin types that shine even with makeup—especially oily skin. Having extra oil is not always terrible because it acts as a seal to protect your skin from losing moisture. But it can be a problem for makeup, so you have a couple of options.

First, you can forgo foundation as a part of your makeup routine. Just use an oil-absorbent powder to blot some of the oil and lessen that shine; then use your powder blush and your eye makeup. You may find this plan works well for you on most days.

If you want to wear foundation, it is a good idea to choose a water-based one. And make it a habit to use your astringent during the day when you feel a buildup of oil on your skin. Put some astringent on a tissue and wipe the length of your nose, the sides of your nostrils, your forehead and your chin. Then reapply foundation and powder if needed.

Disappearing Makeup

Everyone absorbs makeup through the skin, but some people absorb it much faster than others. I call this the "disappearing makeup." I have a friend who swears that before she is ready to go out of her house in the morning, her makeup has disappeared. This happens to some people often and to others only at certain times: during menstruation, during times of stress, when particularly tired, or when dieting.

The instinctive solution for this problem is simply to apply more makeup. Don't! You will only end up with a mask on your face. Rather, put on your regular face and then learn to periodically punch up your makeup. This means occasionally checking your face during the day to see if you need more concealer, a touch more foundation around your nostrils, on your nose or on the top of cheekbones, and/or added powder blush anywhere for a rebirth of color.

So get used to the fact that at certain times in your life this will happen. It doesn't mean that you aren't putting on your makeup in the right way or that you need to apply more; it just means you will need a little extra help throughout the day.

When Contouring Is the Answer

I explained what contouring is (page 75) and how it is used by women to accentuate or minimize some of their features. Now let's take this a step further, and explain how you can use contouring to sculpt your face so that common facial structures that may be unappealing are transformed into pretty illusions. You may want to reread that section to remind yourself how to contour well.

THE WIDE NOSE

Many years ago, when I first learned how to apply makeup, I also learned how to contour my nose. Now I don't do this every day, but it is important for me when I am filming or being photographed because the camera tends to exaggerate my features. I also usually contour when I am going out for the evening.

After I have applied my foundation, I take the contour cream and apply it in two lines down the sides of my nose, on either side of the nostrils, on top of the nostrils and to the tip of the nose. This makes my nose look thinner, and my nostrils look closer together (it gives them sort of a pinched look). Now I blend the cream with my fingertips until the lines disappear, and there is no definition between my regular foundation and the contouring cream. I then take my highlighter or lighter foundation and blend it into the indentation from my nostrils to my mouth to open up and lighten that area.

Now I take my highlighter and draw a narrow line down the center of my nose—from the spot between my eyes to the tip of my nose—and blend it with my fingertips so it disappears. Next powder, and that's it. The illusion is created—I now have a narrow nose.

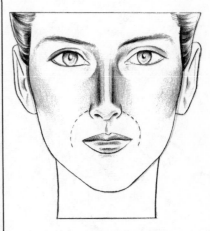

WIDE NOSE

A SHORT, THICK NECK

You'd be surprised at how many actresses use this trick, because swanlike necks are few and far between. I suggest first applying your regular foundation lightly down your neck, almost to where it meets your shoulders. Now use a towel to pat off any excess foundation. Take contour cream or the darker shade of foundation (which can function as a contour cream), mix a little bit with your regular foundation and apply it to either side of your neck.

You have just created the optical illusion of narrowing your neck. Now powder it with a puff and spray with water to set your makeup so that it won't come off on your collar.

A DOUBLE CHIN

Use the darker foundation, mixing a little of it with your regular foundation right in the palm of your hand. Now apply the new color just under the tip of your chin and outward so that it forms a triangle under your chin. Now blend it, stroking away from the chin, with very gentle fingertip strokes. Finish off with translucent powder. This will create a shadow, and will greatly minimize a double chin.

TO EMPHASIZE YOUR CHEEKBONES

This is the most popular use of contouring. To emphasize your cheekbones, take the dark contour and put it at your hairline. Now gently bring it halfway down to just beneath your cheekbone—it should arc and be the shape of a wedge of watermelon. However, if you have a heart-shaped face like mine, rather than deemphasize the heart shape, accentuate it by making your cheekbone line an upside-down watermelon—arc the shadow up, and then down.

If you have full cheeks, apply the contouring shadow under your cheekbone, almost from the temple to the middle of the jaw, and highlight with your lighter foundation on the cheekbone itself.

TO SOFTEN A SQUARE JAW

Shade along the jawline and highlight (with the lighter foundation or a highlighting cream) the center of your chin so that you are bringing more attention to that and not to the outside of your jaw.

TO MAKE A RECEDING CHIN MORE PROMINENT

This is the time to use highlighter on the entire chin and even a little bit under the chin so that it seems to bring the chin out and forward.

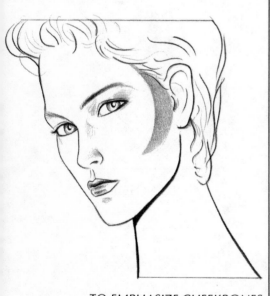

TO EMPHASIZE CHEEKBONES

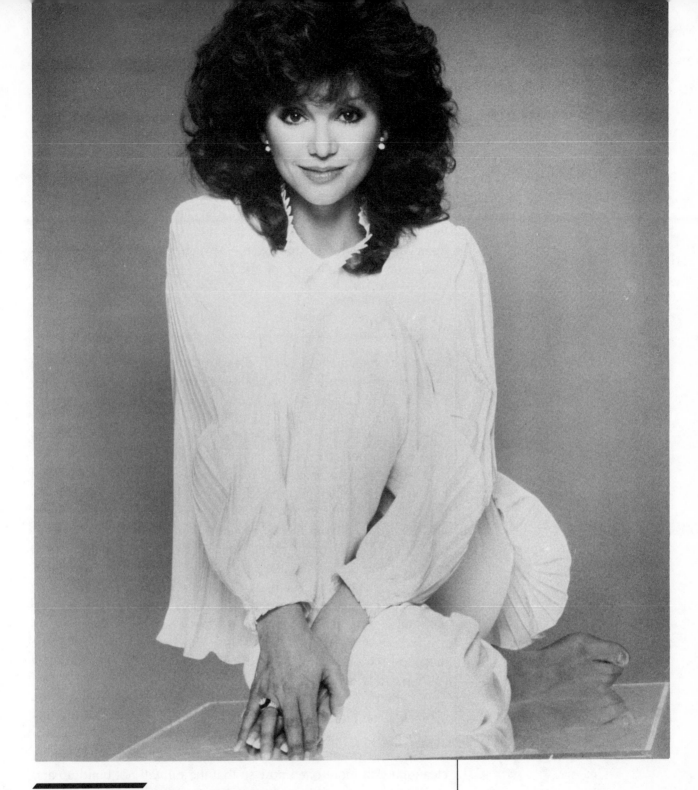

THE OCCASIONALS: DEALING WITH CHANGES

Your makeup routine is a habitual part of your life. You perform the simple ritual every day, adding the additional steps for evening as you like. But some days are not as great as others. As Jean Giraudoux said, "Only the mediocre are always at their best."

In order to enable you to deal with these special conditions as they arise, and to do so comfortably and easily—after all, many of them will happen again and again—here are some tips I have discovered, many of which work for me.

Menstruation

The hormonal changes our bodies go through before and during menstruation affect every part of our lives. Our mood swings have been well publicized. And we know that our skin suddenly develops some strange habits—women whose skin never breaks out wake up with a pimple or two. Women who always look healthy suddenly have complexions that are pale and washed out.

The important thing to understand is that these are natural changes, they are temporary and they may happen every month. So the trick is to learn how to deal with the problems they may create, and then go on to your regular routine.

At these times of the month the color of my skin disappears. I look wan and pallid. To alleviate this, I do not put on more foundation. My skin, though, seems to demand something now, so I take some cream rouge, put it in the palm of my hand, and mix it there with some of my regular foundation. Then I put this new mixture on my face as I would my foundation. The result: Instead of more makeup I have a livelier glow that gives my skin the added color it so desperately needs.

If you don't wear foundation during the day, try this punched-up version on these special days. You may find it will give you the lift you need.

Some skin gets oilier during menstruation. It is important to clean the skin more often now so that the oil will not build up and end up as blackheads (see Chapter 2, page 52). There is nothing you can do to prevent pimples from happening at these times except clean your skin and hope for the best. But these pimples are not tragedies. I have learned to expect them, and when they come I am not aghast, and if they don't I'm pleasantly surprised.

I really believe that most of the time a pimple seems bigger to us than to anyone else, and that no one will notice it. Remember that pimples at this time of month are temporary. They will go away.

Travel

When traveling bring everything you will need to continue your normal makeup routine. Just choose the necessary products (leaving out optionals you probably won't need on the trip), put them in plastic zippered bags (or commercial travel bags made for cosmetics) and off you go.

If you are a terrific planner, you will have collected sample bottles of your cosmetics, so when you need to pack up for a trip, you can take these smaller containers rather than carrying the larger ones. This enables you to take along as many cosmetic products as you want without filling up your whole suitcase.

Many of the tools you will need are already in your makeup bag (see The Perfect Makeup Bag, page 123). But be sure to include for traveling a favorite soap, the shampoo and conditioner of your

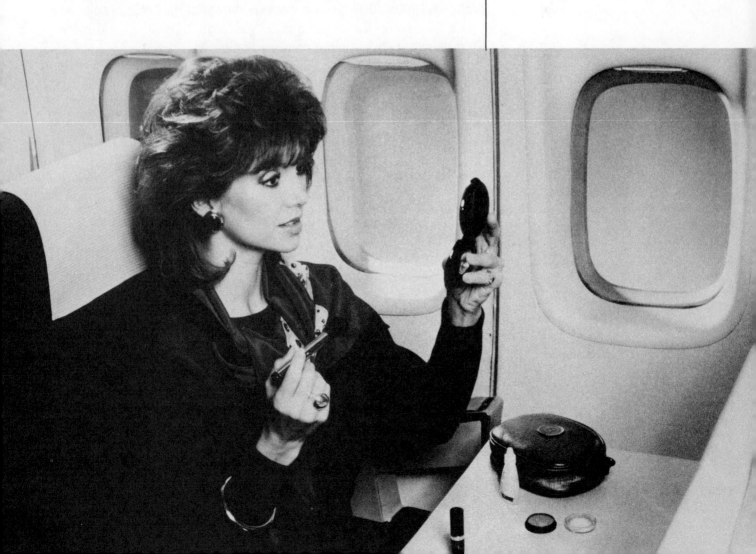

choice, alcohol (especially if you have pierced ears), pads for makeup remover, tissues, a special comb for wet hair, eye drops and perfume. Always bring your baby oil and petroleum jelly—the first is a good moisturizer for your body and a good makeup remover, and the second is an eye gel and lipstick.

Dieting

When you are on a diet, just as when you are under any stress (or are fatigued or premenstrual), your body is in a "different" condition. This will affect your skin and how makeup reacts with your face. Dieting, however carefully and healthfully followed, takes its toll on your body. Your pores will be cleaning themselves, pushing impurities to the surface, and your skin will simply not look its best.

This is the time to follow your makeup and skin routines carefully and religiously. And use the perks—add that cream color to your foundation for an extra glow your skin is missing. Add more blush to your cheeks, your chin, and under your brows.

The oiliness of your skin may change while you are on a diet, so you may have to watch the amount of moisturizer you are using. If your skin is oilier, change from an oil-based foundation to a water-based one. If your skin is drier, use a heavier moisturizer. The important thing is to watch for the changes and be aware that you can alter your makeup routine to fit these temporary times!

A word about crash diets. Don't go on them, ever! Not only are they unhealthy for you, but they will cause havoc with your skin. Drastic changes can make your face fall, and no matter how you try to fix it with makeup, the damage will be visible and difficult to correct. The easiest lesson to learn is not to go on a crash diet in the first place.

Cold Sores

Most cold sores or fever blisters are a type of herpes virus. Approximately 60 percent of all Americans have this kind of herpes. But you can get a cold sore for many other reasons, including emotional stress, intestinal upset, fever or fatigue. Even sun- and windburn can cause these blisters (make yourself a note that sun blocks for both cold and hot weather can work wonders to prevent this type of cold sore.)

Sensitivity to certain foods also tends to set off an outbreak of these fever blisters. The next time you get one, try to figure out if a food could have been the cause, and, if so, then either leave this food out of your diet for a while or at least minimize your intake.

The treatments for cold sores vary. You can dry them with camphor, menthol, boric acid powder, some antiviral medications and zinc oxide. You can also mix some baking powder and alcohol and apply it to the spot. Try these until you find one that works for you. And see a doctor if the sores persist.

If you get a cold sore, don't throw a lot of makeup on it. First try to dry it out with any of the products mentioned above. Then put light foundation on it and leave it at that. If the sore is on the lip, just leave it alone until it goes away. Again, putting more makeup on these sores only calls attention to them. (If you get one of these in your mouth, ask your doctor about using milk of magnesia as a mouthwash—it neutralizes the acid in your mouth and thus helps the sore heal faster.)

THE MAKEUP AREA IN YOUR HOME

Not everyone can have a private makeup area in her home, complete with mirrors and built-in dressers and drawers and the like. But you don't have to have such an elaborate area in which to store your makeup and put it on. It is enough to merely set aside some place that is your very own.

I believe that every woman should have enough consideration for herself to set aside her own special place, no matter how small, where she can make up in private and in peace. It will not only benefit you, it will be a place you will truly enjoy. If you have children, if you have a one-bedroom apartment, if you share a bathroom with every other member of your family, it may not be that easy to find a private corner for yourself. But try—and here are some ideas that might help.

First, find part of a desk, a dressing table, or your bathroom counter (preferably with a drawer) that you can claim as your own.

Now invest in a mirror that you can put on this counter, one with lights on it. There are some that have a magnifying mirror on the other side—you don't need it for making up because it can distort your face, but you may want it to help take care of your skin.

Choose a mirror with lights that illuminate you from above and below. It should have at least four bulbs, either frosted or clear (frosted light gives you a softer look; clear blubs are harsher, but they give a more realistic and natural look). Never use fluorescent lights, or you will always look a little green.

Even if you have this mirror, try to put it next to a window if you have one. Making up near natural light is the best of all.

Decide if you want to make up standing up or sitting, because if you prefer the latter you'll need a comfortable chair.

Claim a drawer—commandeer it if you have to—that is all yours. This is where you will organize all your makeup and skin care products. You can buy plastic organizers in any hardware store. Use them. Put your products and tools in some sort of order that makes sense to you—either by color, by products—all eye products to-gether, all creams together or all colors that match together. You'll need to organize this only once—and then clean the drawer monthly, eliminating products that are no longer fresh. Remember, creams, especially those without any preservatives in them, spoil, just like food. So buy them in small sizes and get rid of them period-ically.

Now get yourself a plastic (so if it falls over, it won't break) eight-ounce cup and fill it with your makeup brushes. Place it on the counter within easy reach of the mirror and your makeup. This makes it easy to get a brush when you need it.

Get a second cup for your hair brushes and combs, and put it next to the other one.

Collect your astringent, your moisturizer and any other creams you own, and, if you can, set them in a drawer because these are the products that suffer most from heat and light changes. In the sum-mer, if your home is very warm, you may want to keep the astrin-gent and creams, and even some eye pencils, in the refrigerator.

In your drawers, keep your cosmetics either in plastic boxes (the kind they make to organize your kitchen drawers) or in plastic, see-through zippered bags that you can take with you when you travel.

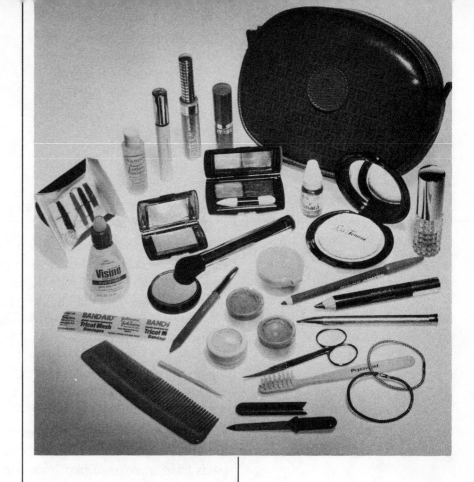

THE PERFECT MAKEUP BAG

I don't believe in anything being perfect, except for my makeup bag. It is. It took me years to make it that way, and now I never leave home without it. Ever. My makeup bag has in it everything I might need when I am not in my home—not only for retouching my face, but for accidents and emergencies of various sorts. I can't tell you how many times I have found myself either on the set of "Dallas," in a restaurant or at a dinner party, when someone next to me needs a Band-Aid, a scissors, thread, glue, a lipstick, a breath freshener— and I just reach into my bag and there it is. I love it whenever someone says, "I wish I had . . ." and I reach into my little bag and there it is. In this way I have converted more people to carrying this wonderful little bag!

The bag itself is made of plastic or leather and is only six inches by three or four inches (it can even be a little smaller, depending on the style you like). A bag this size fits into almost every purse I have, the exception being a tiny evening bag. When I use my evening bags, I always carry my regular makeup bag in my car so I have everything I need not too far away.

As far as what goes into the bag—the following list contains everything I have in it. You are the best judge of what you need. If something I've listed just doesn't fit your needs, leave it out—there is no sense putting something in your bag you will never use.

Make a mental note to clean out your bag once a month, making sure to throw away any makeup that is no longer fresh and anything you really don't use. It's better to throw away something unclean that may contain bacteria than to use it on your skin.

So, here is the perfect makeup bag:

- 1. *Tiny comb*

- 2. *Mirror*

- 3. *Compact of translucent powder:* You can use this pressed powder with the puff it comes with or with a brush. Usually these compacts have a piece of plastic on top of the powder. Don't throw it away. It is there to protect the powder and to separate it from the puff. If the puff that comes with the compact is not made of rubber, buy yourself a tiny rubber one that you can wash easily. Check the mirror. If it is a good one that does not distort your face, then you won't need the other mirror listed above. One is enough.

- 4. *Cream blush:* I usually buy the hypoallergenic kind in a very small plastic case in a basic shade that will look great on me anytime. I use this on my cheekbones, under my brow bones, on my chin—even on my lips—almost anywhere to give me an added healthy glow when I need it.

- 5. *Chlorophyll:* You can buy a tiny bottle of mouth freshener in any drugstore, and because you use so little at a time it will last for a year. I prefer the chlorophyll because it is so concentrated and it has no sugar in it.

- 6. *Contouring base:* Because I have learned how to use contouring in my business, and because I find it a useful tool to use on my face, I always carry a small container of my darkest shade of foundation for contouring touch-ups. If you do not contour your face, leave this out of your makeup bag.

- 7. *Foundation:* I have two small containers of my lightest and my regular shade of foundation, so no matter where I am I can touch up my face (remember that trick for your eyes and lips). If you use only one shade of foundation, just carry that one in a small bottle. Watch for department store giveaways—I often pick up small samples of the foundation I love in order to carry them in my makeup bag.

• 8. *Moisturizer:* Even though it does you no good to put moisturizer on when you already have foundation on your skin, it is a good idea to keep some with you for days when you aren't wearing foundation and your skin will need moisture. It's also great for moisturizing dry hands, and for any other moments when you will need it (it's easier to have it in the bag than to try to remember to put it there on days when you know you will want it). Keep the moisturizer in a tiny plastic container, well sealed. Again, try to pick up a sample size that is small enough to carry around in your bag.

• 9. *Lipstick pencil:* This is for outlining your lips.

• 10. *Lipstick brush:* Just in case I want to use tube lipstick.

• 11. *Lipstick in a wand:* Usually clear or a colored gloss (if you prefer petroleum jelly, carry a small tube).

• 12. *Powder blush:* This is crucial so you can always touch up with color. Remember, use the cream in the morning and touch up during the day with powder. Also remember that you can put some over your eyebrows, on your chin, the tip of your nose, and on your neck for an added glow.

• 13. *Blush brush:* Get a retractable, medium-size brush to use with the blush. Some powder blushes come with brushes in the case; they are fine, but I find a slightly bigger one is better. And remember, it doesn't matter that the brush is bigger, because it retracts and takes up the same room in your purse no matter what size its head.

• 14. *Eye shadow:* A light shade is wonderful to open up the eyes.

• 15. *Mascara*

• 16. *Eyebrow pencil:* This pencil is great for touching up your eyebrows and is terrific for drawing a line in your lower lid, in the corners of your eyes, and for touching up your eye liner. I always buy the kind with a self-sharpening top, so no matter where I am I can sharpen the pencil.

• 17. *Eye pencil:* Use this to touch up your eye liner above and below the eye. This is the soft kind you can smudge.

• 18. *Astringent:* I use it to clean up oil that has accumulated on my nose, my forehead and my chin.

• 19. *Manicure scissors:* For cutting anything.

• 20. *Tweezers:* For tweezing anything.

• 21. *Vitamin E stick:* This looks like a lipstick in a tube and is a wonderful moisturizer for your lips. You can also put it under your eyes if you are not wearing any foundation or concealer.

• 22. *Child-size toothbrush:* This is the most inexpensive and accessible eyebrow brush and eyelash separator you can find.

• 23. *Nail file:* I have a tiny diamond dust one that comes in its own cover so it won't get hurt and won't scratch anything else in the bag.

• 24. *Dental pick and/or dental floss:* I can't imagine being without a dental pick. I use it after each meal, and between as the need arises. The dental picks I have found in drugstores come in their own cases, so they are sanitary and are protected so you can't hurt yourself while searching around in your bag.

• 25. *Ponytail rubber bands (covered):* If you have very short hair, forget this. But with hair like mine, I like to be able to, on the spur of the moment or when the occasion arises, put my hair up away from the face.

• 26. *Pillbox:* I carry my vitamins (they digest better when taken with meals) and any medication necessary.

• 27. *Threads:* In your drugstore, pick up a matchbook or other small case with needles and threads in it.

- 28. *Band-Aid:* I carry just one for emergencies.

- 29. *Atomizer of perfume:* This is wonderful for a pick-me-up of scent.

- 30. *Saline solution:* A small bottle of commercial saline solution does wonders for tired eyes at any time of the day. It soothes safely, and makes your eyes sparkle.

That's it. It may sound like a lot of things, but gather them around, put them into that little bag, and you'll be delighted and surprised at how easily they fit and how efficiently the whole combination of items works. And watch—next time someone mentions they need something and you have it, I bet you'll smile with great satisfaction.

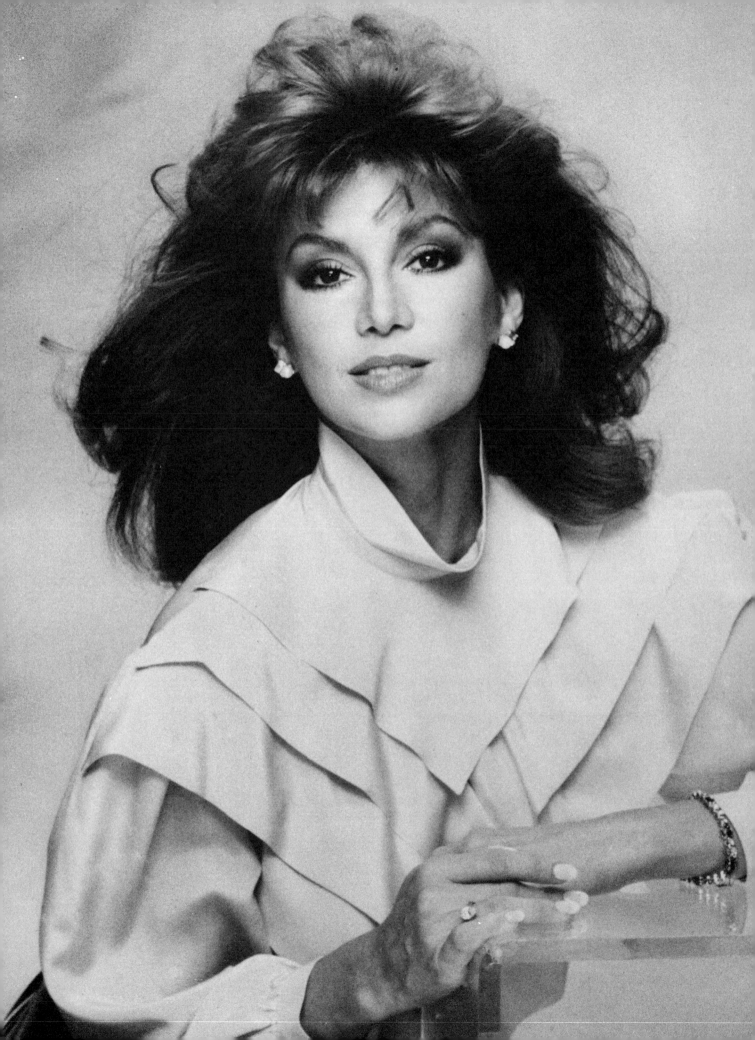

CHAPTER 4

HAIR POWER: THE BEAUTY OF HAIR

THE PRINCIPLES OF HAIR CARE*

Gorgeous, magnificent hair, flattering to your face, touchable to any hands, captures attention and crowns your beauty. Shining, healthy hair, whether it's long or short, thick or thin, blond or black, helps you feel confident and look beautiful. The key words are healthy and flattering—a great hairdo that makes the best of you is a direct result of your care and a hairdresser's good cut. Both will give you the assurance that you look your best. That is *hair power*.

Thus, in this chapter you won't find a series of sketches of perfectly triangular, beautifully heart-shaped and flawless oval faces with suggestions of the categorically ideal hairstyles for those shapes. I don't know many women who have a totally round face or an absolutely triangular one for which someone could advise the perfect hairstyle, and I have never believed that there is such a thing as *the one* "right" hairstyle for a specific shape of face. There are too many

---

* Much of the basic information used in writing this chapter was prepared with the help of Dr. Lee Hunter of Jhirmack Enterprises, Inc., and with Marlene Barnett and Randi Sorenson, also of Jhirmack.

exceptions to the rule (as a matter of fact, I think the exceptions are the rule). When creating a hairstyle for your face, there are *so* many other things to consider—the size of your eyes, the shape of your nose, your cheekbones and your forehead, the texture of your hair, and, of course, your life style. Thus it would be presumptuous to tell you *how* to wear your hair.

The Basic Cut

We begin with the core of hair power, the essence of having a beautiful head of hair—the basic haircut. Now this does not mean that you must find a cut and keep it forever. Rather, a basic cut is flattering to your face, appropriate to your life style and easy to care for but also gives you the flexibility to change the hair*style* to suit your changing needs and moods. We all have many faces—the housekeeper is a mother is a professional is a party guest is a friend is a sometime athlete. Each of us needs a hairstyle that is not time-consuming to create but that can be easily, slightly or dramatically changed to fit any occasion.

Appropriate to your life style is essential here. If you spend most of your time at home, your needs may be different from someone who spends most of her time in an office, or on a construction site, or in a classroom. Each of us needs a hairstyle that fits our job, personality and time constraints. If you have the time for hot rollers and know how to handle a blow dryer, then you can have a hairstyle that demands more in terms of care than someone whose time, skills and/or patience are minimal. Moreover, you may feel like Mata Hari, but if your job is at a desk at a computer company, wearing an exotic, exaggerated and head-turning hairstyle is probably inappropriate. Leave the outrageous for after hours and recognize that you require a hairstyle that can fulfill your dual needs—as a daytime professional as well as a nighttime celebrator.

Your basic cut, then, should be flexible, appropriate, and reflective of your energy, your self-confidence, your attitude about yourself—because that is the image it and you will present to others. How do you get it? Read on.

Choosing a Hairdresser

I love my hairdresser. His name is José Eber, a man who has a talent for creating the perfect hairdo for each of his clients. He took me under his wing ten years ago when my hair was more than a minor disaster, taught me the importance of taking care of my hair, humored my penchant for often changing my hairstyle, and has always given me haircuts that are manageable, flattering and easy to care for. That is what every hairdresser should do for his or her clients. How to find the perfect one for you? Here is my list of do's and don't's in selecting, dealing with and keeping a hairdresser:

1. Find a hairdresser through a personal recommendation. If there is someone you know who has a haircut you admire, or you see someone on a street or at a party with a pretty hairstyle you think may look great on you, ask her where she gets her hair cut. Don't be shy—I have found that women are flattered to be asked and generous with the information.

2. Make an appointment and walk in with confidence. Don't be intimidated by a fancy salon or a preoccupied receptionist. Be gracious but firm; announce your arrival and ask when you may see the hairdresser. If you are kept waiting, ask why. Ask any other questions you like. Remember, hairdressing is a service—you are the client and the priority at any salon should be to serve you.

3. On your first visit, when the receptionist gives you a robe to change into, don't do it. Meet your hairdresser with your hair the way you wear it normally, in the clothes that are yours, so he or she can see the whole you, the image you present. This will help him understand "who" you are and to create a style that will fit you. But this also means that you shouldn't "dress to the hilt" or pretend to be someone you are not. Be yourself—but be your best self.

4. Notice if the hairdresser has the time to talk with you—not only to discuss the style that would be flattering for you (beware if he immediately tells you he knows just the perfect style for you) but also to find out what kind of life you lead, how much time you have to care for your hair, how skilled you are at using some of the tools and what kind of hairstyles you like. All this information will help him to create your hairstyle—so if he doesn't ask, volunteer the information. If he doesn't care—leave immediately.

5. If you see the hairdresser creating the same hairdo for all his customers—watch out. It may be the only one he knows, or he may be the kind who does only one "in" hairdo at a time. A good hairdresser creates an individual style for each of his clients.

6. Once you have chosen a hairdresser, talk to him honestly. Tell him what you like in a hairdo, and what you don't like. I really believe that if you end up with a hairstyle you hate, you must accept some of the responsibility. To avoid such a catastrophe, keep saying to yourself, "It is my hair that's being styled and I have something to say about it!" Any good hairdresser will respect that.

7. Don't skimp on a haircut. The hairdresser you like may be more expensive than others, but if he is really good, it will be worth it. Remember, if you get a cut you hate, you are going to have to put out more money to have somebody else fix it. If you want to save money on a haircut, go to the stylist you like but have him or her cut your hair shorter than usual so you won't have to return as often.

8. A good hairdresser will not make you dependent on him. He will give you a haircut that you will be able to take care of yourself, and he can show you how to do it yourself—so ask him! If you find when you get home that you can do nothing with your hair (and you find that the only person who can is your hairdresser) tell him that the cut isn't right for you. If he doesn't understand, you may need to switch to someone who does.

9. As for waiting for a hairdresser: I always call about thirty minutes before my appointment to find out if he or she is running late. That saves me from having to wait around at the salon.

Now that you have your new hairdresser and your basic cut comes the most important part—caring for your hair. A great cut and an understanding, accommodating and talented hairdresser will mean nothing if your hair is not in good condition. Healthy hair is not a myth or an unattainable goal—anyone can take care of her hair. It is easy, can be inexpensive and the results are (barring any unforeseen disasters or careless techniques) successful and worth it.

Just as in caring for your skin and learning to use makeup, there are tools, terms, techniques and treatments to learn about and to use.

The Tools

As in every care program, you need some basic "tools of the trade" to be properly prepared to nurture your hair.

COMBS

You need a set of good combs—a styling comb; a rattail comb (used both for combing and, with its "tail," for further styling and lifting your hair); and a wide-tooth comb, especially if you have long and/or permed hair—it is used to minimize breakage of hair and split ends. It is also good for distributing conditioners and color evenly (keep one in your shower). Some of you may want a pick, which is used to lift a hairstyle, to comb curly or permed hair and to remove tangles from long hair. Preferably combs should be made of hard rubber—most plastic combs have sharp edges that can cause damage to the hair.

BRUSHES

You need at least three brushes—one natural-bristle, synthetic or plastic brush used for brushing out hair when it is dry; one round brush which adds curl to your hair while you blow it dry; a third is a small version of the natural-bristle brush to carry in your purse. You should know that a natural-bristle brush is best for gentleness to your hair. When you brush your hair, do it thoroughly but softly—don't pull. Remember, a hair in the head is worth two in the brush!

BLOW DRYER

A blow dryer is a must! For many of us, the days when we sat under a hair dryer for two hours—rollers in place, waiting for our hair to curl and dry—are gone. The blow dryer dries hair quickly and at the same time allows you to style it into an easy, natural look. Blowers can be purchased in different drying powers (from 850 to 1500 watts). Many also have several settings and speeds of air temperature and air flow. It is best to use a dryer that is about 1000 watts because excessive heat will overheat and overdry your hair and scalp. But I think it's useless to have low- and high-watt dryers—get a higher one and set it low. You can get an attachment to your dryer called a *diffuser*—it fits on the end and spreads and scatters the heat to dry permed or naturally curly hair.

Here are some hints I have learned over the years on how to best use a blow dryer:

• Keep the dryer on the low-heat setting. This will minimize overdrying of your hair and scalp while drying your hair uniformly.

• Always hold the dryer at least six inches away from your hair.

• Keep the dryer moving—don't leave it on one spot for a long time.

• Dry the back of your hair first, then move toward the front.

• If you want more fullness to your hair, put your head down and blow-dry until it's slightly damp. Now throw your head back and finish styling.

• If you are using a round brush, put the hair around it smoothly and don't pull—or the hair will break.

HOT ROLLERS

Hot rollers are a wonderful invention! When I was in high school, it took me hours to set my hair in rollers (sometimes on empty frozen orange juice cans) and then sit under the dryer. Now I just roll up my hair in hot rollers, wait ten minutes—and I'm done. How do they work? Each roller contains a waxlike substance in the center that becomes heated and retains the heat long enough to curl the hair. Using hot rollers on dry hair produces terrific bounce and curl. Some hints on using hot rollers:

• Use end papers whenever you can to prevent the ends of your hair from splitting.

• Remember the size of the roller will determine the size of your curl, and that the longer you keep the curlers in, the tighter the curl will be.

• When you remove the rollers, don't pull, or the hair will tangle and break.

• Make sure the rollers are cool before you take them out (this will give you a better set).

CURLING IRONS

Curling irons are optional and can burn and otherwise damage your hair unless you know what you are doing and do it carefully. They come in many sizes—the size of the rod determines the size of the curl. There are several different kinds: the *marcel* (used mainly by professional hairdressers), where the handles are held together to keep your hair in place as you roll it; the *spring iron,* which holds the hair in the iron as you roll it; the *crimper,* a flat iron with very small wave patterns (the waves make your hair zigzaggy, kind of frizzy); and the *hot comb,* which will straighten curly hair. Some tips:

- Never use an iron on wet or damp hair.

- Don't hold it for too long or you will burn your hair.

- Don't put too much hair in it at once. You have to be patient and just take small sections at a time.

END PAPERS
These are tiny and thin rectangular papers to fold on the ends of your hair before you use hot rollers. They prevent the ends of your hair from splitting.

ROLLERS
If you prefer to use a cap dryer or to let your hair dry naturally, you may want to first set your hair in rollers. If you sleep in rollers (I hope you sleep alone), use the soft ones made of sponge.

HAIR SPRAY
Hair spray is made of polymeric resins, aerosol and nonaerosol, which keep your hair in place. They come scented and unscented (I prefer the latter so the fragrance won't interfere with my perfume). It used to be that hair spray made hair look stiff and untouchable. But today's sprays leave your hair soft and pretty. Aerosol spray gives best results in terms of a good "hold" with a minimum amount of resin on your hair (that's because it has a fine mist and even distribution). Always hold the hair spray container at least six inches from your hair to avoid wet spots.

The Terms

pH
This refers to the amount of hydrogen in a solution, such as shampoo. It determines if a solution is acid or alkaline. The amount of hydrogen is measured on the "pH scale" (0 to 14). A shampoo that

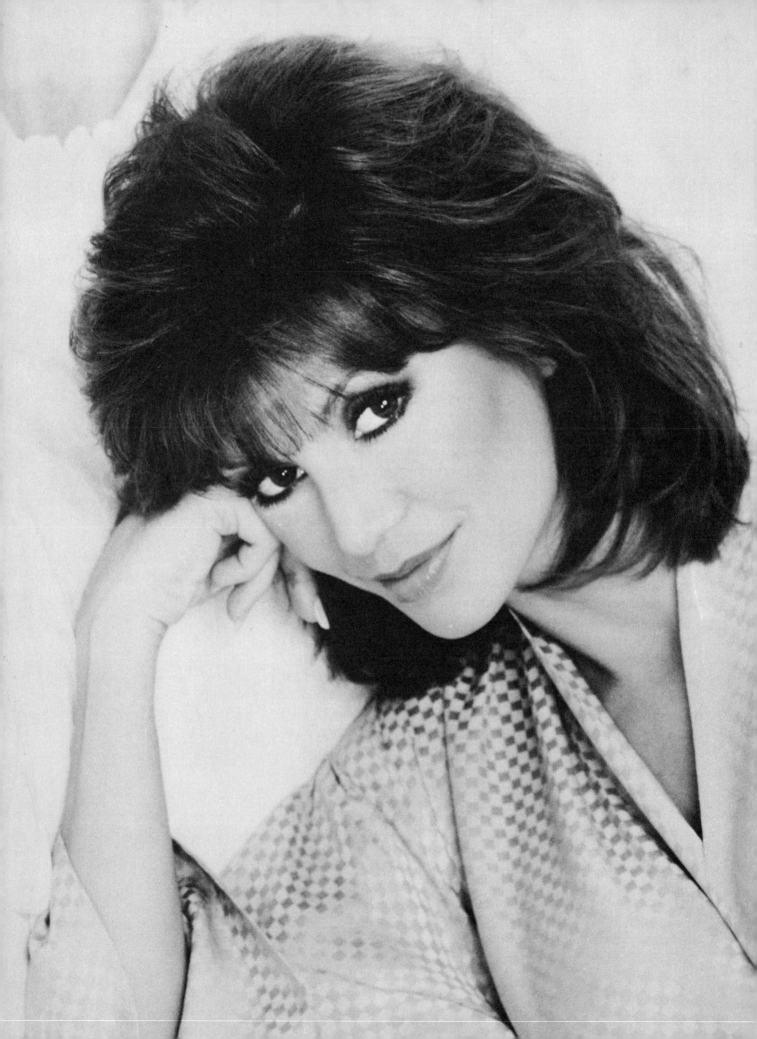

is acidic will register from 0 to 6.9 on the scale; 7.1 or above is an alkaline shampoo, and 7.0 is neutral (the amount of alkaline and acid is equal).

What does all this mean? The pH of a shampoo affects the pH of your skin and your hair—the higher the pH of the shampoo, the more alkaline it is, and therefore the more damaging to your hair (it will dry it). An acid-balanced shampoo has the same pH as your skin and your hair and will not damage either (it won't change the pH). If you use a high-pH shampoo, experts advise to follow it with an acid rinse.

SHAMPOO

• *Plain shampoo:* Used on hair in good condition. It usually contains a soap or detergent (and is thus alkaline on the pH scale). If you have tinted, lightened or damaged hair, don't use this shampoo.

• *Nonstripping shampoo:* For hair that has been permanently colored (it removes the least amount of color from your hair). It is an acid shampoo, mild on the hair, and usually has a conditioner in it. It can also be used on dry or damaged hair.

• *Acid-balanced shampoo:* Has the same pH as hair and skin, and can be used on all types of hair.

• *Medicated shampoo:* Contains ingredients designed to correct certain scalp or hair conditions. It is often prescribed by a doctor. Be sure to follow the directions carefully.

• *Antidandruff shampoo:* Usually contains a special ingredient to counteract dandruff formation and a conditioner mixed with a plain shampoo. There are several types available for either a dry or an oily scalp. When using this shampoo, again follow the manufacturer's directions. Be sure to vigorously massage your scalp and to rinse thoroughly to remove all traces of the dandruff.

• *Egg shampoo:* Recommended for very dry, brittle or overlightened hair. It can be bought or made at home (add a whole egg to a nonstripping shampoo). When using an egg shampoo, rinse your hair with cool or lukewarm water; if you use hot water, the egg will congeal in your hair.

• *Conditioning shampoo:* Contains animal or vegetable additives to correct certain defects in the hair. *Coating* conditioners (usually made of oil or animal fat) will be removed in the next shampoo. *Penetrating* conditioners (containing proteins) will often last through several shampoos. It is true that some shampoos may cause a buildup of conditioners on your hair. The solution is to switch to a less conditioning shampoo for a while.

CONDITIONERS

• *Instant conditioners:* Do not penetrate the hair shaft. They contain a vegetable oil (like balsam) or an animal substance (such as cholesterol). They are left on the hair for up to five minutes and must be rinsed off (they also help in detangling). This kind of conditioner makes your hair look better and feel softer but does very little to strengthen it.

• *Penetrating conditioners:* Contain many different ingredients—animal proteins, nucleic acids, vitamins and oils. This type of conditioner penetrates the hair to help bond damaged fibers; it is left on the hair from ten to twenty minutes and usually lasts through several shampoos. Included in this group are hot-oil treatments, which add lots of shine and body to the hair.

HAIR RINSES

• *Creme rinse:* Used after you shampoo as your *last* rinse. It will soften your hair, give it a shine and make it easier to comb. A creme rinse is really the same thing as an instant conditioner (it just has a different name).

• *Vinegar rinse:* Separates the hair, dissolves the soap and gives hair brightness and softness.

• *Lemon rinse:* Has some lightening quality and is effective on blond hair.

• *Color rinse:* A prepared rinse that is used to highlight or add temporary color to your hair. This rinse remains on the hair until the next shampoo.

SETTING AIDS

• *Setting lotion:* A liquid containing a polymeric resin to give body to the hair before you blow it dry or set it in rollers. It helps your hair keep the set. Some also contain conditioners.

• *Gels:* These are thick, used for roller sets, blow-drying your hair and to give your hair the wet look. Some gels come with color in them.

• *Thermal styling lotion:* Used to help set your hair when you blow it dry. It contains a conditioner to protect the hair from the heat.

• *Mousse (foam):* Used with roller sets, blow dryers and to get the wet look, adding sheen, manageability and body.

Types of Hair

FINE HAIR

You've seen this kind of hair—it hangs limply on the sides, is flat on the top and is lifeless. Some people call it "baby hair." It tends to be flyaway and is difficult to style. The best tip for this kind of hair, besides getting the right cut, is to use a penetrating conditioning shampoo with extra body as often as you like (hair seems to look fuller after a shampoo), a ten-minute conditioner every other week (it will give it more body), and no products for oily hair. If your hair and scalp also happen to be oily, more frequent shampooing with an "extra body" conditioning shampoo is a good idea.

THIN HAIR

If you have this type of hair, you know it! It is sparse (you can see your scalp through it), fragile and breaks easily—so handle it gingerly. You need an acid-balanced shampoo, to be used only once a week or so. Creme rinses may untangle your hair, but they will also keep it looking limp. You can use special body conditioners to add fullness to this type of hair.

COARSE HAIR

Coarse hair is usually difficult to control because it tends to be thick and wiry. It is healthy hair, but on humid days, it can get out of hand. If it isn't dry, it may help you to wash it every other day or even every day with any normal shampoo. Frequent haircuts can do a lot to keep coarse hair under control.

THICK HAIR
This hair can be fine, it can be coarse—but whatever it is, you have an abundance of it, and I wouldn't complain if I were you. You should choose a shampoo that fits the condition of your hair—dry, oily or normal. Any rinses or conditioners are fine. Do condition—this will untangle your hair, and you'll need it!

DRY HAIR
Easily identifiable, dry hair looks and feels like straw, is usually split at the ends and is very dull and lifeless. Generally you are not born with dry hair—you make it dry. Any hair that has been bleached, permed or straightened will be dry. It needs a lot of care—oil treatments, acidic shampoos (and don't wash it every day or it may get even drier), and conditioners full of moisturizing ingredients such as proteins. (Those of us who color our hair should know that the process damages only the hair the chemicals touched—new growth will again be healthy. Miraculous, isn't it?)

OILY HAIR
Unless freshly washed, oily hair always looks greasy, as if you've slicked it down with gel. It always seems to look dirty. It is limp and stays close to your head, refusing to have any body. Moreover, having oily hair usually also means you have an oily scalp. You need to shampoo often with a shampoo especially made for oily hair, taking care to cleanse the scalp thoroughly with a double application of the shampoo. Don't use a conditioner except on the ends (and then only if you have to)—or you'll end up with "oilier" looking hair. If you need to use a detangling instant conditioner after shampooing, choose an extra-body product which is low in oily conditioners.

NORMAL HAIR
Normal hair is the envy of all of us—the head of hair you always wanted—shiny, full of body and absolutely gorgeous! Lucky you, you can do whatever you damn please—wash, condition, anytime and as often as you want—because whatever it is you're doing, it must be right. But do remember, abuse it and you may be envying someone else.

TECHNIQUES FOR HAIR CARE

There are many things you can do to your hair to change it. But the key to successful changes is to understand the process and to undertake it in the correct manner. Here are the various techniques and tips on how to do them right.

Shampooing

Equally important as skin care in your beauty routine is shampooing. If you were only to do one thing for your hair, shampooing it the right way and with the shampoo geared specifically for your hair would be it. It's not just that clean hair is prettier. Experts warn that unless your scalp and hair are cleansed regularly, the buildup of perspiration and oils will be a perfect breeding ground for bacteria. How many times a week you should shampoo is up to you—you should pay attention and see how often your hair and scalp feel dirty. Most hairdressers will tell you that generally oily hair needs to be washed more often than dry or normal hair. But if you have some knowledge of what kind of hair you have, how often it gets dirty, and if you use the shampoos and conditioners for your hair type, you really can be the best judge of how often to wash your hair.

Shampooing is a process we all need to understand, because all too often we've learned how to do it as children and thus have not reeducated ourselves as to how to shampoo properly.

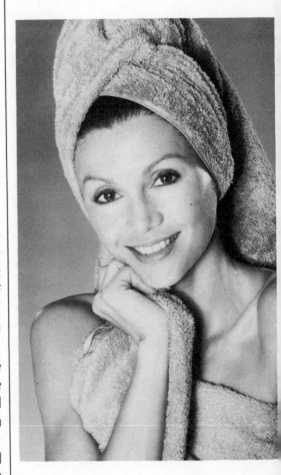

HOW TO SHAMPOO

Start your shampoo with warm water, rinsing the hair until it is completely soaked (not just damp). Use a soft stream of water—a hard stream of water can break off your hair at the roots. Put a *small* amount of shampoo in your hands and rub to make a small lather. (If you use too much shampoo, it will leave your hair *extra* dry, especially if your hair has been bleached.) Now put this on your hair and massage, rubbing back and forth. (You need to rub it into the hair and scalp thoroughly in order to loosen the dirt and grease. If you don't get a good lather, just add more shampoo.) Never use your nails!

If you feel you need it, wash your hair again—but this time use only half the amount of shampoo. When the lather is thick and your hair seems to have soaked it up, rinse thoroughly, time and time again, rubbing your hair to make sure the water reaches everywhere and all the dirt and shampoo are flushed out, especially at the base of the neck. Test the water running out of your hair; when it is clear, your hair is clean. Now use your conditioner, leaving it on as long as the directions advise. Then rinse with cool water to close the pores on your scalp and make your hair shiny. If you're done rinsing, do it one more time anyway. When you *are* done, pat your hair with a towel—don't rub it (I have found that rubbing just knots and breaks hair, especially if your hair is thin, damaged or fragile).

Permanents

I, too, have had a permanent—haven't we all? I did it because I felt I needed a change—and I loved it for a while (I'm not sure those around me were so thrilled!). It gave me the lift I needed.

It used to be that getting a permanent meant ending up with very curly hair, period. But, just as other hair care techniques have changed, so have permanents. The following can be done at home, or you can have your hairdresser do them for you:

BODY PERM

A body perm gives your hair fullness and volume but no curl. It is wonderful for straight hair that needs body, limp hair that just won't take a set and for those of us who prefer not setting our hair in hot rollers every morning. The body perm makes hair more manageable.

MEDIUM-CURL PERM

In this procedure the hair is wrapped on medium-sized rods, resulting in firm curls which give your set a stronger and longer-lasting hold.

THE WASH-AND-WEAR PERM

This kind of perm gives you a tight curl, so you can wash your hair, let it dry by itself (or dry it with a blow dryer with a diffuser attachment), and you're ready to face the day. Don't use a hot blow dryer or a hairbrush on this perm. When I had my perm, I often just washed my hair and used my fingers to continuously fluff it up as it dried naturally. Another hint: With this hairstyle, whenever I was in a hurry, all I had to do was lightly spray my hair with water and let it dry—it looked like a new, just-done hairstyle!

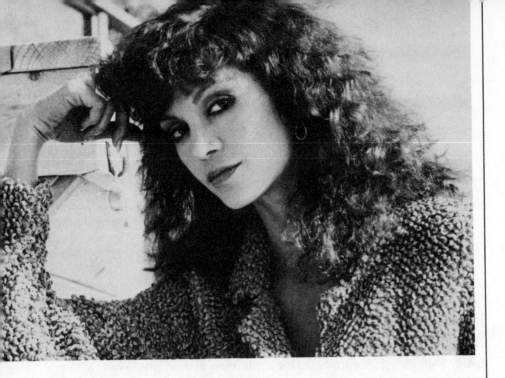

ROOT PERM

This is a fairly new procedure where only the hair at the scalp is permed. This makes the hair look thicker and healthier, while the ends stay unpermed and pretty. (But you must consider that, eventually, your roots will be your ends!)

THE HOME PERM

Always choose a home perm that is made for your hair type. If you have frosted, bleached, color-treated or any damaged hair, please do a test curl before you start, or ask your hairdresser if he or she thinks your hair can stand a perm (also ask about perm safety if you have henna or any metallic dye on your hair—most likely you should not perm if you do). Be sure to read and follow the directions carefully on any packaged home permanent kit. Here are some added tips from Dr. Lee Hunter at Jhirmack:

1. Collect your tools, including the rod size for your hairstyle (tiny for tight curls, larger for a looser curl), a rattail comb, clips, cotton, end papers, a spray bottle, a plastic bag, a timer, a protective cream for the hairline and rubber gloves.

2. Start by lightly washing your hair. Be careful not to scratch your scalp or it may later burn from the perm solution.

3. Never wrap your own hair. Have someone do it for you. The wrap is the most important step. Make sure the ends are straight and flat inside the end papers. The right amount of uniform tension in the wrap is extremely important because too much tension will cause damage and breakage and too little tension will result in a weak curl.

4. Make sure the rods are not rolled too tight against the scalp

or the plastic fasteners will cause a crimp in the hair which can result in breakage.

5. If your hair is dry by the time you put in the last rod, spray it lightly with water before applying the wave solution.

6. Follow the manufacturer's instructions for timing your type of hair. Apply the neutralizer.

7. Remove the rods gently, and, with the neutralizer still on your hair, massage your head for a minute and then rinse well. Make your final rinse a cool one.

8. Don't shampoo for forty-eight hours.

9. Remember: *You now have processed hair.* You will need to change your shampoo and conditioner to ones that have been formulated for your hair.

10. Use a deep conditioner at least once a month.

11. Always use a wide-tooth comb or a pick (not a brush) when combing wet, permed hair—you'll avoid breakage and split ends.

12. Always use an instant conditioner or creme rinse after shampooing in order to avoid combing damage.

13. If you use a hair dryer, use it on the lowest setting, and/or with a diffuser.

Straightening

Straightening, or relaxing, is a chemical process by which your curly hair is permanently straightened. There are two kinds of "hair relaxers"—one is very strong (it has a pH of 12) and the other one (the Thio relaxer) is milder and can be done at home. Ask your hairdresser about both. Once you have straightened your hair, you'll need to use an acid-balanced shampoo and a good moisturizing conditioner. You should note that tinted, lightened and other processed hair should not be straightened.

Hair Coloring

I have been coloring my hair for years. It adds glow to my hair and gives it more body. Hair color can improve the appearance of your hair by adding shine and sparkle, covering the gray, and enhancing your skin coloring. For hair that is very fine and limp, the hair-coloring process will add body.

There are several types of color that can be used, from a one-time color that can be shampooed out to the permanent tint. Here is a brief description of the varieties available.

TEMPORARY

Most temporary hair products come as hair rinses. Temporary colors do not penetrate, and thus will not produce a dramatic change in your color, but they will add highlights or intensify your own color. They wash out completely with one shampooing (that's why they're called temporary!). Temporary coloring is usually made from acid dyes approved for food, drug and cosmetic use by the FDA, so no patch test is required. If, however, you choose a package that calls for a test, be sure to do it.

SEMIPERMANENT

Semipermanent color lasts through four to six shampoos, but each time the hair is shampooed, the color fades gradually. These formulas do not contain peroxide and won't change the hair structure. You can use semipermanent colors to conceal gray hair without changing your natural color.

PERMANENT

This type of product is exactly what it says: permanent! It will remain on the hair until it grows out or is cut off. The only way it can be altered is to use chemicals that strip the dye from the hair (like bleach). There are three types of permanent hair color:

• 1. *Vegetable:* The most popular is Egyptian henna, made of all natural ingredients. If applied properly, your hair will have lots of shine and body along with beautiful highlights. A few precautions should be observed when using henna: Never perm hair that has been treated with henna—mild disaster could occur when trying to use both. Also, it is a very messy paste and if splashed around, the spots will stain.

• 2. *Metallic:* Known as a color restorer, this forms a metallic coating over the hair shaft. Never perm, tint or lighten hair that has been treated with a metallic dye. Hair treated with metallic dyes is usually dry and dull in appearance. (Often the hair will have a greenish, purple or pinkish cast.)

• 3. *Synthetic permanent tint:* Most hair color is done with synthetic permanent tint, where the dye or tint is mixed with hydrogen peroxide. This makes the color permanent—it will not wash out! These tints usually may be applied over hair that has been permanently waved, but you should wait at least two weeks and do a strand test before your color. You should also do a patch test before using this type of tint. Permanent tints can be used to completely cover gray, lighten or darken hair or intensify your natural color. Special effects such as *frosting* and *streaking* are most commonly done with bleach to lighten the hair, then a tint or toner applied to the bleached hair. *Frosting* is done by placing a transparent plastic cap over your hair, after which small strands of hair are pulled through holes in the cap and then bleached or colored. With the technique of *foil wrapping,* strands of hair are covered with bleach and then wrapped in individual pieces of aluminum foil. By applying heat to the foil (usually by sitting under a hair dryer) you accelerate the bleaching action in your hair. You may notice that throughout this procedure you resemble a creature from outer space—but it's worth it. A newer technique is *hair painting,* which gives a terrific effect of many subtle colors in your hair. Here your hairdresser "paints" bleach or tint on the hair with a brush anywhere you want the color.

THE PATCH TEST
When using a permanent tint, a predisposition, or patch test must be done twenty-four hours before applying color to check if you are allergic to the product. This test must be used each time, even though you may have used the same product for years. This is a very important process—it could avoid many problems!

The procedure for giving yourself this reaction test:

1. Select a small area on the hairline behind your ear.

2. Clean it gently with mild soapy water. Pat dry, but don't rub your skin.

3. Mix one-quarter teaspoon of color with one-quarter tea-

spoon of peroxide, and mix well. Using a cotton swab, dab a small amount of color behind your ear.

4. Let it dry. Leave uncovered for twenty-four hours, then examine your skin for any redness or irritation. If any itching occurs or an irritation appears, don't use this product—you may be allergic to it.

HOME HAIR COLORING
The basic procedure for at-home hair coloring:

1. Assemble the tools you will need, including plastic gloves, a protective cape—try an old towel—for your shoulders (also, put down a newspaper or an old sheet to protect the floor), a wide-tooth comb, a plastic applicator bottle (if not provided by the manufacturer), and petroleum jelly or heavy cream to protect your hairline from the stain.

2. Shampoo your hair only if it has a heavy buildup of hair spray or if it has not been shampooed for some time (if shampooing is necessary, it is best to do it twenty-four hours before coloring hair, giving your scalp a very light massage so you won't scratch it). Always apply the color to dry hair. If your hair is tangled, comb it, keeping the comb away from scalp. Never apply tint if your scalp has abrasions, cuts, open sores or any signs of disease.

3. Put on the towel and gloves. Apply the protective cream all around your hairline, making sure not to get cream on your hair. Mix the color according to the manufacturer's instructions. Start coloring at the so-called "most resistant area," where the hair is lightest if darkening with color, or where the hair is darkest if lightening with color. Cover the root or regrowth area first. Follow the instructions for timing on the root area and then proceed as directed.

4. Rinse and shampoo your hair, then follow with a good conditioner suited to your hair type.

LASH AND BROW TINTING
This is great for lashes and brows that are blond or light brown. Tinting is done with a special dye designed to be used around your eyes. Never use a dye that is used on the hair—it could cause severe eye damage. The gentle tint for eyelashes and brows works the same

way permanent tints work. A very low volume of peroxide is mixed with the tint, applied to the lashes or brows, left on for ten to fifteen minutes (I usually wipe a bit off with tissue to see if the color is the shade I like), then gently washed off with warm water and nontear shampoo. The color will last six to eight weeks. You will love it because you'll need little or no mascara.

Hair Removal

SHAVING

You can shave using a safety razor or any electric razor. Never use soap when shaving with a safety razor as it is very drying—use a shaving cream (or a gel with a conditioner in it) followed by a moisturizer to reduce chances of irritation. If you want to shave around your bikini line, try using baby oil—it's a model's trick for quick depilation with no rash.

TWEEZING

This is a temporary method of removing the hair around the eyebrows. Apply a warm pad to the area for thirty seconds before tweezing. Remember to always clean your tweezers with alcohol or astringent and to tweeze in the direction the hair grows. When you finish, use your astringent on the area.

DEPILATORIES

Depilatories are designed to remove hair by dissolving the hair shaft or by adhering to the hair shaft and pulling the hair from the skin surface as the depilatory is removed. They can be classified into two distinct groups: physical and chemical. The two most common *physical depilatories,* wax preparations and honey preparations, are applied to the skin surface after they have been warmed. A small piece of muslin cloth is then pressed over the wax; when cool, the muslin is pulled away from the growth pattern. When the wax or honey is removed from the skin surface, it takes any hair found in that area along with it. Always read and follow the manufacturer's directions when using these products.

Chemical depilatories remove hair by completely dissolving the hair shaft at the surface of the skin so it easily washes off. Always read and follow the directions; many people can be sensitive to these products, so do yourself a favor and do the patch test. Also, some chemical depilatories, even though safe, can feel as if they are burning the skin. I have found a remedy: Take an equal amount of the depilatory and zinc oxide (a cream you can buy in any drugstore without a prescription) and use this mixture—it really prevents burning. After removing it, put an antibacteria cream on the area (like Neosporin, available without a prescription at any drugstore, or Aloe Vera cream). Then put facial moisturizer on the area. One word of caution: Never use a depilatory on the face or breasts because that skin is too fragile. Use a product specifically designed for facial skin.

CHANGING CONDITIONS AND YOUR HAIR

Special and changing conditions can affect your hair. Learning about the relationship between nutrition and hair, weather and hair, and the effect special problems can have on your hair will help you deal with these changes.

Nutrition

We feed our bodies, and that food affects not only our general physical health but our skin and hair as well. How direct is the relationship between nutrition and hair? Experts say that, since the average scalp grows hair half an inch a month (if it were only one hair growing, it would grow 250 feet in one day!), normal hair growth requires a constant supply of nourishment. The food we eat is the primary source of nutrition, and it is the fuel required to "drive" the living cells. If we don't eat enough nutritious food, then our hair will also be deprived of nourishment. As a matter of fact, some doctors use the condition of your hair as a symptomatic measure of other conditions—for example, hair loss may be a sign of anemia, and both hair loss and dandruff could be a sign of stress. Moreover, thin and sparse hair could be a result of a vitamin and mineral deficiency. We are what we eat!

This means, first of all, eating well-balanced meals—that seems to always be the answer, doesn't it? But it's so for a reason. If you eat well, the results will show on your body and in your hair. And if you

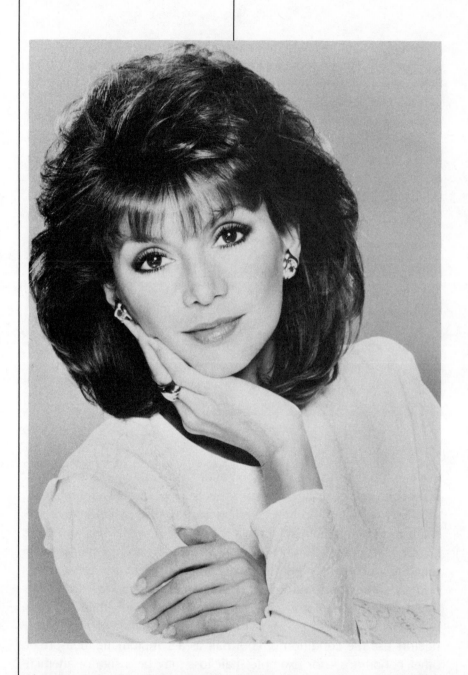

abuse your body—these results will also show, and you won't like them. For example, a lack of iodine can lead to a thinning and loss of hair. You also need sulfur (available in foods with high-quality protein, such as meat, fish, eggs and milk) for proper hair growth. Balanced meals means just that—foods with vitamins, minerals, proteins and plenty of water. Hair needs a constant supply of good proteins in the diet—this is not an option but a must! Remember, you can condition hair from the outside, but you must also nourish it from the inside. So minimize the no-no's (foods high in sugar, fat and processed chemicals) and emphasize the nutritious (those high in proteins, natural carbohydrates, vitamins and water). For further information on a well-balanced diet, you may want to refer to the diet chapter in *The Body Principal*.

And a reminder one more time—never ever go on a crash diet! Besides ruining your health, it is terrible for your skin and your hair. Don't do it!

Seasonal Changes

Climates change, and with each coming of winter or summer, the elements affect the condition of your hair, which in turn can affect how you style it.

The sun damages your hair. It's a fact, and there's no getting around it. But I can't tell you to stay out of the sun—I don't believe in self-deprivation! I love the sun, as long as I am protected from its harmful effects. I have learned that you can *care* for your hair and *protect* it while you are in the sun by remembering the following tips:

1. When you go out in the sun, wear a hat or scarf. If you don't like either, at least put some sunscreen on the part in your hair.

2. There are "hair sunscreens" on the market—conditioning creams that will cover and protect hair from the sun's drying rays. I apply oil or a deep conditioner and leave it on while I'm sunbathing, swimming or playing volleyball, and then I shampoo my hair. It works great—not only do I protect my hair, but I also condition it at the same time.

3. If heat and humidity have taken the life out of your hair, you may want to get a body perm for the summer. If not, you may want to do what I do—use both a milder conditioner in the summer (so it won't be so soft) plus a setting lotion or gel to give your hair more body.

4. I often wear my hair up in the summer. It looks great with hats; it's easier to keep conditioned; it's less exposed to the sun; and it's versatile enough so I can go from pool to dinner with no fuss.

Wearing it up also means I damage it less—no styling with a blow dryer and no hot rollers.

5. I always put a moisturizer on my hair before I go in a pool or in the ocean. Remember—hair with salt water dries out quicker, so your hair must be protected from the ocean.

6. Condition, condition, condition in the heat of the summer (and in the freezing winter, too).

Winter is not much kinder to your hair. Wind and cold air attack relentlessly every year, and they'll keep doing it, so the best and easiest solution is to keep your hair covered outdoors (for the skiers among you—headbands don't count! Get a warm hat that covers your hair and your ears—if you can, get a ski mask that will protect your skin, too). Also, dry, indoor heat robs your hair of needed moisture, so conditioning is the answer. For flyaway hair, try rubbing some hair conditioning cream in your hands and then spreading it lightly on your hair.

Occasional Problems

DANDRUFF
According to Dr. Lee Hunter, dandruff is excessive scaling of the scalp without clinical signs of inflammation. The diagnosis can be made with your eyes—you can see the flakes. (If the flakes were caused by psoriasis or a type of dermatitis, you'd be able to see signs of infection on your scalp.) Dandruff can start early; many infants have such "scalp scaling." But most dandruff starts at puberty and intensifies gradually over the years. Incidence of dandruff is usually greater during the winter months because of the dry conditions. The solution is often as simple as shampooing with a dandruff shampoo (be sure to wash the *scalp* well, too). Frequent shampooing with a conditioning shampoo can sometimes help control dandruff.

HAIR LOSS
If you sometimes find hair on your brush or in the drain in the shower, this is normal. Your hair grows in cycles; it falls out naturally and is constantly being replaced. But sometimes hair loss can be a symptom of other problems (besides nutrition). If your hair is falling out in clumps, or bunches, there may be a medical reason. Some

hair loss is attributed to anemia, to diabetes, and to other diseases, so see your doctor if the condition persists. Other causes of hair loss are more or less controllable—if you take too many drugs, if you're under a lot of stress, if you're addicted to crash diets, you may lose your hair. An answer may be to live a life of moderation, to eat well-balanced meals, and to take care of your hair. If you've just had a baby, don't worry because hair loss is common after pregnancy.

To treat hair that is fragile and thinning, the experts at Jhirmack suggest the following:

1. Sleep well, eat well-balanced meals and exercise. This will start you off to a healthier life style.

2. See a doctor—if there is a medical reason for the hair loss, he or she can treat it. Ask about your vitamin intake.

3. Wash your hair with a gentle massage and with an extra-body shampoo for thin, damaged hair.

4. Don't wear ponytails; don't use hot rollers—these can only further break and pull out your hair.

5. Don't color or perm your hair until it grows back nice and healthy. If your hair has really been thinned out, you may want to wear a wig while you're treating the problem.

Wigs

There are times when you may want or need to wear a wig. Those of us in films often wear wigs for different parts we play. But I truly recommend that you wear one only if you need to because of serious hair problems. Not only does a wig prevent your scalp from breathing, it flattens your own hair. Cheap wigs are no good at all and should be avoided. If you need to wear one, invest in a good quality, natural-looking wig, and follow these tips:

1. Pick a wig that fits your facial coloring and is not too different in color from your real hair (unless you need it to play Cleopatra!).

2. Buy one at a reputable salon and have it styled there just as if you were having your own hair done. (It's very common to just drop off a wig, do your errands, and return for your new "do.")

3. Make sure the wig is well made (that the hair is not thin and that it allows some air through so your scalp won't suffocate).

4. Wash your wig with shampoo—not with a detergent.

5. Treat it as you would your own hair and it should last.

A LIFETIME OF HAIR CARE

Taking care of your hair is a must. It's as essential to a beautiful you as is conscientious skin care and careful, flattering makeup. You've seen how easy it is and how immediate the results. Now all you have to do is—practice. If you follow the hair care advice I have set out, you'll be able to take care of your own hair to make it as beautiful as it can be. As a final touch, then, here is a list of "hair care tips"—the "do's" that will ensure you do the best you can for your hair:

1. The key to a well-groomed, low-maintenance hairstyle is a good professional cut. If it is financially difficult to get a cut every six to eight weeks, have the hairdresser cut your style slightly shorter. This way you can get ten to twelve weeks from your cut.

2. Shop around for a hairdresser you can trust. Make an appointment for a consultation before you have the cut.

3. If you want to have a perm but don't know how you'll look, try one of the new "wash out" perm kits first. If your hair is colored, check with your hairdresser before attempting *any* permanent.

4. When using hot rollers, use end papers to protect the ends of your hair from damage.

5. Baking soda mixed with water removes hair spray buildup. Baking soda also helps cut heavy scalp and hair odor.

6. Hot rollers are very popular for a quick and easy set. The longer the rollers are left in, the more curl you will receive. Always remember to allow the hair to cool completely before brushing.

7. Most important for a good permanent wave is the proper technique in applying the right amount of tension when rolling your hair on the rods.

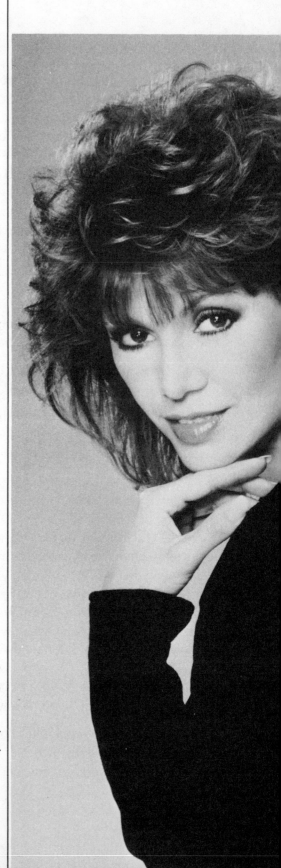

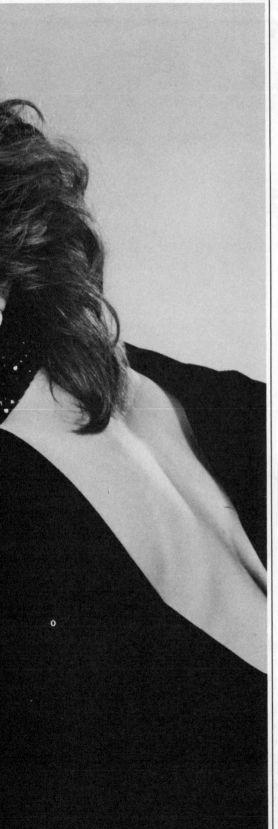

8. Blow-dry hair on a warm setting rather than a hot one, directing hair in a downward motion.

9. When spending the day in the sun, apply a deep conditioner to your hair before going out. You will protect your hair and give yourself a deep conditioning all at once. Cover your hair when you are in the sun to protect your scalp.

10. Always shampoo after swimming and apply a conditioner.

11. If you need to freshen up a natural or curly style, dilute some conditioner in a spray bottle full of water. Use a conditioner that adds a lot of shine. You'll freshen droopy curls and do a "mini" conditioning all at once.

12. Assemble a hair care emergency kit. Depending on your hairstyle, you could include: a travel curling iron, hair spray, decorative combs, a covered rubber band, travel-size hot rollers, "spritzing bottle" (refillable, trial-size hair spray bottles are great), gel and bobby pins.

13. Keep a wide-tooth comb in the shower to comb through ends. Never use a brush on wet hair.

14. Apply a deep conditioner when doing your housework, watching TV or reading.

15. Keep combs and brushes clean. This aids in keeping your hair fresh at all times. Weekly brush and comb baths are a must. Wash them in shampoo—if it's good enough for your hair, it's certainly good enough for those brushes.

16. Make sure your hair is dry before using a curling iron or hot rollers.

17. To add body, hold your head down and blow-dry. This will add a lot of fullness.

18. Excessive use of any product causes oily hair.

19. Proper manipulation when shampooing (use the balls of your fingertips, not your nails) aids in healthy scalp and hair.

20. Treat your hair gently, as if it were fragile. This will insure that your hair will stay as healthy as possible.

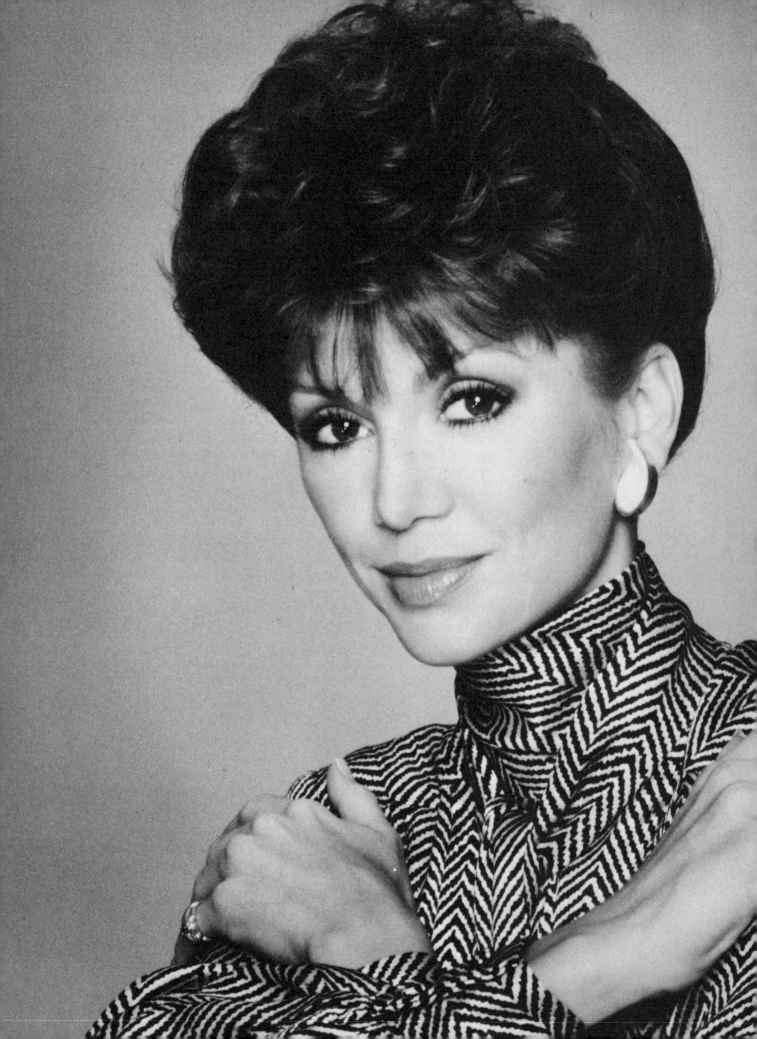

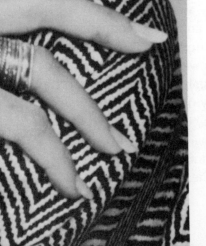

CHAPTER 5

HORMONES, YOUR BODY AND BEAUTY

Feeling beautiful involves attaining harmony between how you feel and how you look. If you take care of the outer you—care for your skin, learn to apply makeup that brings out the best in you, wear a hairstyle that is flattering, appropriate and easy to manage—and if you pay attention to your physical and emotional needs, you will feel and look as beautiful as you can.

But there are times when something is askew; when monthly turmoil seems to affect everything you do. There have been many times during my life when my emotional reactions and my physical discomfort have puzzled me. For years I was bewildered by the occasional erratic and unpredictable seesawing of my emotions, by uncomfortable and sometimes painful physical symptoms in my body, and by seemingly mysterious fluctuations in sexual desire. Such mercurial feelings and symptoms perplexed and baffled me, and the common explanation for them—"Oh, you must be getting your period"—seemed to be simplistic. I was aware that premenstrual behavior was known to affect women in different and sometimes inexplicable ways. But such a matter-of-fact response seemed inadequate for what can be a serious problem.

As I talked to my women friends, I discovered that we share this commonality of fluctuations in physical and emotional well-being, and also in the waxing and waning of our sexuality. Further discussions with doctors resulted in the somehow comforting finding that there are physiological and medical reasons for these changes. Dr. Sandra Aronberg, a gynecologist and obstetrician practicing in Beverly Hills, California (who is attending physician at Cedars-Sinai Medical Center in Los Angeles and a clinical instructor of obstetrics and gynecology at the University of California, Los Angeles), explains, ''Our ability to function in our daily life is tied to two factors: One is our hormonal system, and the other our emotional state—our self-image, including our feelings of being desirable and beautiful. We are now finding that realizing and maintaining such a sense of self, which we can strengthen by taking better care of our bodies, is something we can do for ourselves. We are also finding that, even though we have little control over the symptoms that the fluctuations in our hormonal system cause (which have a direct effect on our emotional behavior, our physical wellness, our sexuality and our beauty), we can recognize and come to terms with them and their effect on our lives, and try to alleviate them.''

It is important and reassuring to understand that it is such hormonal activity which can explain seemingly irregular behavior and oscillating emotions, definite physical changes in the body and fluctuating sexual feelings, and that between 30 to 80 percent of the women in the world routinely experience such powerful and disturbing symptoms. The enormousness of the incidence of such symptoms has promoted research and studies resulting in the findings that these women are suffering from what has been termed premenstrual syndrome (PMS).

PMS is a monthly occurrence of clinical symptoms that can cause havoc in your life, particularly if they are misunderstood and if they paralyze you so that you have difficulty functioning. According to Dr. Aronberg, ''These often severe symptoms, which are caused by physical changes due to the rise and fall of hormones or to hormonal imbalance between levels of estrogen and progesterone in the body, occur regularly from one to two weeks prior to the onset of menstruation (they do not include menstrual cramps or discomfort from bleeding). Such symptoms include any or all of the following: water retention and weight gain, headaches, unexplained and fluctuating emotional changes (including sexual desire), cravings for sweets and salt, hot flashes, depression, painful joints, swollen and painful breasts, great fatigue, backaches, acne, and more.''

Now not everyone who experiences some of these symptoms is suffering from PMS. "But," says Dr. Aronberg, "if you chart your menstruation and the occurrence of such symptoms and find that they happen with some regularity and some degree of severity each month, you are probably a woman who has PMS."

DEALING WITH HORMONAL CHANGES

The news is actually good news—because once you know that this often called "crazy" or "neurotic" behavior is not crazy at all but is due to a physiological condition, you can make a conscious decision to try to deal with the symptoms and not let them control your life. Here are some suggestions:

1. Accept that you suffer from some degree of PMS and realize you are not alone. Recognize the symptoms and expect them, because reducing your anxiety may alleviate them. Doctors believe that a positive attitude will help you deal with the symptoms and remove the control they have on your life.

2. See a doctor. If he or she is unsympathetic or doesn't show an understanding of PMS, get another doctor. Ask about the medications available for relief of some of the symptoms. Ask about the advisability of vitamin therapy—some researchers believe that a high dosage of vitamins B_6 and E helps you relax and may alleviate some of the symptoms.

3. Watch your diet. Eat well-balanced meals (they seem to be the answer to almost everything, don't they?). Watch for cravings for salt (which can lead to water retention and bloating) and for sweets. Fill up on foods with proteins and long-chain carbohydrates—not candy bars but foods that give you energy over a long period of time. Try eating some natural diuretics—like parsley and watermelon, and drink diluted iced tea. Stay away from caffeine (particularly in coffee but also in strong tea, cola and chocolate)—it can increase breast tenderness and seems to have an adverse effect on many PMS sufferers. Be aware that the effect of alcohol greatly increases when you

are premenstrual, and particularly if you suffer from PMS (it enters the bloodstream faster than at other times; if you normally drink two glasses of wine, one may now make you drunk).

4. If your breasts are sore at this time, be sure to wear a bra. The support will minimize some of that pain. Reduce any activity that causes extra movement to your breasts (like running). And don't drink caffeine.

5. Talk to other women. I am often amazed at how little information some women share about physical and emotional symptoms they experience and about their sexual problems or questions. Don't be afraid of boring your friend—it's probably the only time you can be sure you won't. Don't feel uncomfortable when asking her about her premenstrual problems and/or about the waxing and waning of her sexual desire—and, in turn, don't be judgmental, competitive or dishonest when another woman asks the same of you. I believe we have a lot to share and a lot to learn from one another.

6. Exercise—here I go again, right? Well, listen to Dr. Aronberg: "There are some findings that athletes and people who are in good shape physically seem to have fewer problems with PMS. Exercise really seems to help—it's a great way to alleviate many of the symptoms." It may be particularly helpful for those women who experience a dwindling desire for sexual activity, because it has been shown that if you increase the blood flow to the vaginal area, it swells in a manner similar to when you are sexually aroused. Thus by working out you can almost trigger your body into forgetting its uncomfortable state and concentrate instead on the pleasure of sexual activity. So develop a program of exercise that fits your needs and does not exert too much pressure on those parts of the body that are painful at this time. Do relaxation techniques—any meditation or slow breathing will help you relieve the tension that so often accompanies PMS.

7. If you develop acne (this is due to the increase of estrogen and progesterone in your system) treat it locally (see Chapter 2, Special Skin Problems). And remember, such skin problems are temporary. Aida Thibiant recommends that you clean your skin more thoroughly and more often to prevent blackheads.

8. At ovulation, the acid-based balance of the vagina changes. Explains Dr. Aronberg, "The vagina seems to be readying itself to

accommodate the sperm. Because sperm won't live in an acid environment, the area becomes more alkaline—you will find that the mucus in the vagina is runnier and clearer (in order for the sperm to penetrate, the mucus has to become thinner)." After ovulation, during the time when PMS may occur, some women recount that their entire body seems to give off a different scent. Be aware that this is normal.

9. You may experience some temperature change in your body —right before ovulation your body temperature drops, and at the time of ovulation (when PMS begins) your body temperature will rise.

Sexual Fluctuations

"Less intelligent animals," says Dr. Aronberg, "are sexually active only when they are fertile, when they are ready to conceive. But humans have the ability to have sexual relations any time, as long as they are able to function *and* as long as they have the *desire* to do so. And, indeed, most human beings enjoy sexual relations throughout the menstrual cycle, for the pleasure, not just for reproduction." Continues Dr. Aronberg: "A large factor that influences our desire for sexual activity (and probably the most important sexual organ of all) is between our ears—the mind. Sexual desire is largely mental; thus if the mental attitude is affected, so is the sexual desire."

But there are many factors that affect the increase and decrease of sexual desire. One is the changing balance of the hormones estrogen and progesterone in your body. Taking any medication for PMS may also change your desire for sexual relations. Actually, many medications can do that, including hypertension pills, tranquilizers, narcotics and alcohol. (As a matter of fact, it is a common misconception that alcohol heightens sexual desire. Not so. Explains Dr. Aronberg: "Alcohol may lower your inhibitions. It may make you less shy, less introverted and temporarily more gregarious and flirtatious. But physical responses are reduced when you drink, and can disappear completely when you are drunk.") And although some drugs can temporarily heighten sexual response, most—particularly narcotics—dull the senses, besides being dangerous to your health.

Another factor that can affect sexual desire may surprise you— women can also have a decrease in sexual response and desire when they ovulate because of a fear of pregnancy (remember, a large part of sexual desire is *mental*). "Many women, when they know they are ovulating and are more likely to conceive, may not be as relaxed as at other times and may thus be sexually disinterested," explains Dr. Aronberg. "There are other women, however, who are in sexual overdrive during ovulation—their sexual responses are at their peak. Some of this information is puzzling; although we have some knowledge that women who are worried about getting pregnant may have lower sexual desire, there have been no studies showing that these women enjoy making love more at this time if they are secure in their method of contraception or if they cannot conceive. There is no question that these fluctuations involving ovulation exist, but the intensity and the incidence of occurrence differ from woman to woman." Being aware of and expecting such changes in your feelings of sexuality will help you deal with them. So will knowing that they are temporary. It's not broken; it will come back.

Another reason for sexual waxing and waning may be stress caused by PMS itself or by any other outside factors that affect your life. Again, Dr. Aronberg: "Anxiety and tension about the havoc these hormonal changes cause in your life also affect your desire to make love. It is so important to understand that it is these physiological changes that may cause the stress that is affecting such desire."

Remember, also, that other forms of stress may affect your sexuality. (Let me emphasize that this is not related to romance, atmosphere, sexual communication with your partner, mutual attraction, sexual capabilities and the like. The assumption is that all these exist.) For example, concern about various problems in your life can spill over into your sexual relationship. If you are preoccupied with financial worries, office problems or family crises, the resulting stress may curb or restrict your sexual desire. It is hard for most of us to feel relaxed, unwound, unhurried and sexually aroused if we are agonizing about money, if we are unusually apprehensive about job security, or enormously anxious about our children.

There are many techniques designed to alleviate these kinds of stress. Some, like psychological counseling, assist by helping you deal with the problems. Others, like biofeedback, help you learn to control your anxiety so that you can deal with your daily life. Still others, like exercise and a self-care program to make you look and feel better, help you channel such stress out of your system by encouraging you to concentrate on the fitness and beauty of your body, which in turn give you renewed confidence and energy and alleviate sexual tension and disinterest. The important thing to remember is that such stress-related sexual apathy is temporary—when the stress is relieved, sexual desire returns.

One more word about the monthly changing feelings of sexuality. Dr. Aronberg: "After the PMS period is over, you start menstruating, and some women, especially those who have felt a diminished sexual desire during PMS, may experience a rise during menstruation. That's fine—it's an old wives' tale that you can't make love during menstruation. Also note that after your period is over, you may experience a loss of sexual desire because there is a fairly rapid drop in progesterone at this time."

Thus the desire to make love may fluctuate almost constantly throughout the month. During PMS, you may feel a decrease in your desire, followed by an increase during menstruation, and another decrease after menstruation is over. Or your pattern may be the reverse. No matter what it is—be aware that such waxing and waning of sexuality is normal.

Beauty and the Beast

The beast of PMS, of any hormonal changes that so directly and powerfully affect our lives, is tameable. Identify it, realize that it is a normal condition and bring it under your control, and your life will be much more peaceful and pleasurable every month. I also believe in the old adage that the better you look, the better you will feel. Taking care of your body will help you deal with the symptoms of these hormonal changes and will make you look and feel better throughout this trying time. We spoke about exercise and its benefits. Adhering to your daily beauty program will also help. Taking care of your skin, wearing more blush for color and paying attention to your hairstyle and its condition will all make you look better, feel better and thus will help you stay in better shape to deal with this monthly havoc. Spend extra time on yourself, because if your self-image is improved, you will be in a better frame of mind and less likely to let the stress and the symptoms control you.

CHAPTER 6

PLASTIC SURGERY

Establishing a beauty regimen involving skin and hair care, makeup routines and taking care of your inner self, is not enough for everyone. There are many women who are not happy with one or more of their facial or body features, who try to hide them or to otherwise compensate for such feelings of inadequacy. For these women, there is an option: plastic surgery. Each year, thousands of women (and men) undergo cosmetic surgery to alter features they consider dissatisfying; they do so to improve their looks and to gain a feeling of self-worth that has otherwise eluded them. In addition, there are many of us who, as we grow older, may consider plastic surgery as an option to retard and remove the signs of aging that seem to be inevitable.

Plastic surgery is divided into two general categories: reconstructive surgery and cosmetic surgery. *Reconstructive surgery* is usually nonelective surgery; it is performed to correct a person's abnormal feature or condition and make it, as closely as possible, a normal one. Patients who have such surgery include those who have been injured and disfigured in accidents, those with birth defects and cancer patients. *Cosmetic surgery* is elective surgery that enhances a feature of a normal person to make her look better. Such procedures include face-lifts, eyelid surgery and most breast and nasal surgeries.

According to Dr. Harry Glassman, a plastic and reconstructive surgeon practicing in Beverly Hills, California, the only reason to have cosmetic plastic surgery is to feel better about yourself. Explains Dr. Glassman: "People come to my office and ask, 'Do I need to have my face done?' Well, no one *needs* to have a face-lift. It is more a question of "wanting" rather than "needing"; provided she is in good health and a good candidate, surgery can be considered. The only justification for doing plastic surgery is to improve the patient's self-esteem, to improve the way the patient feels about herself—in other words, for herself and herself alone."

Cosmetic plastic surgery is an option that gives a woman a chance to make herself look better or prettier, by either changing a feature she thinks of as a compromise or reversing various signs of aging. It is ideal for a woman who does not want to go through her entire life feeling inadequate about a particular feature she considers unattractive. It can be a solution for a woman who feels that she would be more beautiful if she corrected a problem that is disturbing to her. It may be the answer for someone who has an appropriate, realistic and honest motivation to make herself look better.

There are many things plastic surgery cannot do. It will not transform your life from an unhappy one to a perfect one (unless you honestly attribute such unhappiness to the wrinkles around your eyes or to a crooked nose)—it can only make you feel better about yourself so that your outlook on life may improve. It will not create a totally "new" you—only a prettier one. It will not make you look like your favorite movie star, or fix an unhappy relationship—it is a surgical solution to a cosmetic problem. It will not eradicate or compensate for a lifetime of abuse to your face and/or your body—it can only remove *some* of the wrinkles, only take off *some* of those years.

Understanding such limitations is a prerequisite to being a good candidate for plastic surgery. Explains Dr. Glassman: "People must have realistic expectations about plastic surgery. If you expect it to change your life, don't do it. The patient with a great degree of anxiety over a small cosmetic defect is a poor emotional risk. Conversely, someone who is minimally to moderately disturbed regarding a considerable defect or deformity will most likely be pleased."

Knowing the risks is another prerequisite to deciding to have plastic surgery. Besides the emotional risk of having unrealistic expectations, of feeling guilty about undertaking what some may consider to be "an undue preoccupation with vanity," of spending money on something that is really for you and you alone, there are medical risks that go hand in hand with any surgery. And make no mistake about it, plastic surgery is just what it says—surgery. Explains Dr. Glassman: "Plastic surgery is not like getting your hair cut. While it offers wonderful benefits in that it can make a woman look better and thus feel better about herself, it is still surgery, often major surgery, and should not be taken lightly. But surgical risks vary from operation to operation and depend on the physical condition of the patient.

"If you are healthy, and your expectations are realistic, your motivations sound, and your understanding of the limitations absolute and clear, plastic surgery may be the ideal solution for you, because what plastic surgery does it does in an almost wondrous way."

CHOOSING A PLASTIC SURGEON

A good plastic surgeon is, in many ways, an artist. To be sure, he or she is a medical doctor, a skilled surgeon, trained to heal the body's wounds. He is a "psychiatrist," experienced in probing for reasons and reassuring patients about their inadequacies and anxieties. But unlike other medical doctors, the plastic surgeon is also creating and re-creating visible parts of the body, making aesthetic judgments that will forever affect the patient's precious individuality—her looks.

You and Your Plastic Surgeon

Here are Dr. Glassman's suggestions on choosing a plastic surgeon and on being prepared so that you can establish a relationship based on mutual confidence and trust:

1. To begin, you can get medical recommendations from your family physician or another doctor within the local medical community. You can check with the American Society of Plastic and Reconstructive Surgery referral service (but note that it won't differentiate between a level A and level C surgeon—it will only wean out

the level F's). But the best way to pick a plastic surgeon is to be familiar with his or her work through a personal referral by someone who has used this doctor for plastic surgery. If you know two or three people on whom a certain plastic surgeon has operated, and you like the results, that is probably the best indication that you are in the hands of someone you can consider to be good, someone you can trust. You should know that a good plastic surgeon will probably not tell you who his patients were because he would consider that to be an invasion of those patients' privacy. So you have to start out with someone who has had the surgery and is willing to tell you about it.

2. When you get the name of a plastic surgeon, meet with him and check out his credentials to find out what kind of training he has had. No surgeon should be insulted or offended by that question—if he is offended, get out of his office—and no patient should be intimidated to ask it. The point of such a question and such research is to make sure that the surgeon has completed his training in plastic surgery. The American medical system permits a doctor who has finished his internship to open a practice in whatever specialty he wishes. For example, a doctor need not have trained in neurosurgery to call himself a neurosurgeon—all he has to be is a licensed physician. Such a doctor is not violating any law if he opens an office and calls himself Dr. Jones, neurosurgeon. It is thus important to make sure that the doctor has completed his training in plastic surgery as his specialty.

3. Assess the surgeon as a person. You can't tell everything about a person when you are only starting a relationship, but some basic judgments can be made. Does he find time to answer your questions? Is he kind, considerate, gentle—or is he a prima donna? Does he have an earnest interest in helping you or is he doing you a great favor by consenting to be your doctor? Does he listen or is he preoccupied and hurried? Does he ask you for your desires and your motivations or does he tell you what should be done? And does he seem to like his work or does he ache to be on the golf course?

Take the time to evaluate your doctor—and don't feel funny about it. Your are entitled to a doctor who has the time, the talent and the consideration for you.

4. Be prepared to tell the plastic surgeon what it is that you

want to change—what you want to look like. The more definite your idea, the easier it will be for him to understand your expectations. If you want, you can bring in a photograph of a feature on another person, a feature you admire, to give him an idea of what you aesthetically like. On the other hand, beware of a surgeon who shows you photographs of his work to illustrate what he has done. Remember, he won't show you his complications or his failures—only his great successes.

5. Meet with the surgeon more than once. If he wants to see you once and then operate, find someone else. Any good plastic surgeon should be more than willing, even insistent, on discussing your motives (Is it your mother who hates your nose? Is your husband having an affair with a woman who has breasts larger than yours?), your medical history, and the limitations and probable results of the procedure. If he is a good plastic surgeon he will explain things like the inevitability of scars, the medical risks, the recovery time and possible aftereffects.

6. Educate yourself about plastic surgery so you are familiar with some of the terms and at least have a superficial knowledge about some of the new procedures. Ask about your particular interests—whether it's chemical peels versus collagen or the advisability of using lasers to remove birthmarks. The more information you have, the more intelligent discussions you can have with your doctor, and thus the better decisions you both can make. Ask about the options. For example, if you are considering breast augmentation, the plastic surgeon should tell you about the alternatives for where to put the scars (in the end this may be his choice to make, but you should be aware of the alternatives). If your problem is truly minor, he may dissuade you from having any plastic surgery at this time.

7. Ask about all costs—how many office visits does the price include? If one or both of you are not satisfied with the results, will he redo the work without any additional expense to you? Does he require payment up front? Most reconstructive surgery is covered by medical insurance, but cosmetic surgery is generally not covered (unless your policy specifically provides for such surgery) and can easily run into thousands of dollars. It is better to know the financial expectations from the start.

PLASTIC SURGERY— THE OPTIONS

Cosmetic Surgery Related to Aging

The following types of plastic surgery procedures can correct some of the natural consequences of the aging process.

EYELID SURGERY (BLEPHAROPLASTY)
There are three procedures that can be done to the eyelid:

• 1. *Removing excess skin from the upper lids:* This surgery takes about an hour, and recuperation takes about seven days, after which you resume your normal activities. However, you should wait three weeks before returning a full athletic schedule, because the bouncing and straining can lead to swelling in the face and can precipitate bleeding. The scar in this procedure falls in the folds of the upper eyelid, so it can hardly be seen.

• 2. *Removing fat, or bags, from under the eyes:* This surgery also takes about an hour. It is a very common, precise and successful operation that is done on people of all ages, from teenagers who have a family history of bags under the eyes to middle-aged people who don't want to constantly look tired and sad. This inconspicuous scar is usually in the lower eyelid, right underneath the eyelashes, made from one end of the eye to the other.

• 3. *Removing wrinkles from the lower eyelids:* Dr. Glassman, for one, believes that there is a real limitation regarding the removal of wrinkles under and around the eyes—if a surgeon pulls on the skin too tightly to try to remove every wrinkle, he can distort the shape of the eyes. So, in most cases, the lines will be decreased, but they won't be completely erased. This is an added argument for staying out of the sun (the major cause of most eye wrinkles) and for moisturizing the skin around the eyes.

If wrinkles around the eyes are your problem, you might also consider two other options in plastic surgery—the use of collagen injections or a chemical peel.

FACE-LIFT SURGERY

As we get older, our facial skin loses its elasticity, and, because of the pull of gravity, it stretches. Excess skin accumulates in the folds between the nose and the mouth (called the nasolabial folds), along the border of the jaw and in the neck. A face-lift will make you look as well rested and as refreshed as possible, but it won't get rid of all your wrinkles. You will still have lines on your cheeks, around the mouth and around the forehead (that's fine—you don't want a tight, expressionless face!).

A face-lift is major surgery, taking three to four hours to perform. In a face-lift, the surgeon may go through three steps—sculpting away the excess fat, suturing or tightening the neck and facial muscle system, and pulling and removing the excess skin. First, incisions are made in inconspicuous places (in the scalp, inside the ear and in the back of the ear), and the skin of the face is separated from the rest of the face, exposing the deeper structures. Fat is removed from the desired areas and the facial muscles are tightened and sutured. Then the skin is pulled and placed under tension. The surgeon must take care not to distort the patient's natural expression.

Recuperation from a face-lift takes several weeks.

COLLAGEN TREATMENTS

Collagen is the predominant protein in our skin. Injecting it into humans to smooth away wrinkles and acne scars seems to also stimulate the body to manufacture its own new collagen in places where it had stopped. This use of animal collagen was seen as a great breakthrough because before collagen plastic surgeons used silicone to fill in facial depressions (wrinkles). But silicone has several drawbacks. It is a foreign substance, not a protein like collagen. Silicone injections have resulted in some people developing scarring, inflammation and lumps. Also, it has the capacity to move—it can work its way into the body's lymphatic system and/or into the bloodstream and can later be found in some distant organs (the kidneys, liver, and so on).

Collagen, on the other hand, does not move. Its drawbacks seem manageable, at least as far as its short history shows. For example, although some people can develop lumps from collagen at the site of the injection, they do go away with time. Some patients have also developed inflammations as a reaction to collagen; but such an allergy can now be determined by a simple skin test performed at least three to four weeks prior to having the substance injected. Collagen only lasts for about eighteen months, after which it has to be reinjected.

Dr. Glassman adds an additional cautionary note about collagen: Even though it seems to be an effective natural substance, it is still early in its use to be sure of its total effectiveness. Explains Dr. Glassman: "I would feel better if we had been using it for thirty years. This is not to say that collagen *will* be dangerous, but every new substance should be used with due caution."

CHEMICAL PEEL

This procedure is another way to remove wrinkles. It is especially effective on blond, blue-eyed women with fair skin and fine lines around their faces because they are less likely to develop pigmentation problems.

A chemical peel involves the application of a caustic substance to the skin which causes the skin to burn. It removes the outer layers of skin and relies on the deeper layers to resurface to the top (that is the normal action of the skin—to rebuild new layers). The advantage of a chemical peel is that it lasts longer than collagen (it can last for ten years). However, it has other drawbacks. The recuperation from a chemical peel is lengthy. Your face scabs, so you won't be going out publicly for two or three weeks (whereas after a collagen injection you can go back to work the next day). Chemical peels can depigment your skin (change its color); they can change the body's ability to tan and can leave a very clear demarcation line where the chemical peel stops and where the untreated skin begins. Moreover, peels don't help acne scars (whereas collagen does).

Cosmetic Surgery Unrelated to Aging

THE NOSE JOB (RHINOPLASTY)

This is an operation to either improve the patient's appearance or her breathing capabilities, or both. The wonder of this type of surgery is that it is performed internally (all the incisions are done inside the nose) and therefore there are no scars.

This is the most common of all plastic surgeries and the most technically demanding and difficult to perform. Because the surgery is done internally, it relies on the skin's ability to change when its underlying support changes. So when the surgeon lifts up the skin, changes the shape of your bone and the shape of the cartilage on the nose, at the end he has to redrape this new nose with your existing skin. This makes a woman with thin skin the best candidate for this type of surgery. A person with very thick, oily skin should know that this is a limiting factor because that skin does not always comply with the changes the surgeon has made.

Surgical techniques today make most surgery on the nose successful. Explains Dr. Glassman: "The operation has changed a lot in the last five to eight years. Prior to that time, all surgeons were doing was reducing parts, making the nose smaller. If you came in with a big nose, you had a good chance at having a successful rhinoplasty because the surgeon only had to make it smaller. But now we have recognized that there are many situations in which the patient needs parts of the nose enlarged to fit her face. For instance, take a person who has a big bump on her nose but who has a very small tip. In order for her to have a straight nose, the surgeon would previously have had to remove so much of the nose that the result would have been a tiny nose. Today we would take down some of the bridge of that nose and build up the tip so that the nose and face would be in proportion."

A "nose job" necessitates keeping bandages on the nose for about a week after the surgery. After the second week, almost all the swelling goes down, but the whole recuperation process (for all the swelling to disappear) takes four to six months. In other words, you can expect to look well in two to three weeks, but you won't see the final result for four to six months.

A word about the swelling in plastic surgery, especially in nasal surgery. Again, Dr. Glassman: "Technically, the procedure in this type of surgery necessitates a deliberate trauma to the nose. The patient's bone is actually broken using a hammer and a chisel. It is a controlled trauma, resulting in swelling and bruising, or being black and blue. But there are several things that have changed this uncomfortable and unattractive side effect of plastic surgery on the nose. One is that most good surgeons have become less heavy handed and perform the surgery in a more delicate manner. Second, some surgeons have found that giving patients high doses of vitamins for a week before and a week after the surgery results in less swelling and less bruising. And third, plastic surgeons have found that giving the patient low oral doses of cortisone has resulted in less swelling. The benefits of cortisone in this instance were discovered when patients who were in car accidents, who sustained both head and facial injuries, were given cortisone to prevent swelling of the brain. Plastic surgeons, operating to correct their facial problems, noticed that these patients did not swell and bruise as would have been expected. Now many plastic surgeons routinely give their patients cortisone."

THE EAR JOB (OTOPLASTY)
This is an operation to pin back prominent, protruding ears. It is done by making incisions in the back of the ears, reshaping the cartilage with stitches and then sewing the ears back. It is often done to children after the age of six, and to both men and women at any age. It takes about the same time to perform as a nose job. The ears are then bandaged for about a week after the surgery, and stay swollen for another week.

BREAST SURGERY
There are three types of plastic surgery for breasts—breast augmentation (enlargement), breast reduction and the lifting of the breast:

• 1. *Breast augmentation:* The average woman who wants this operation is in her thirties, has had two children and has suffered some loss of volume of her breasts as a result of those pregnancies. Women see this change right away—their bathing suits and bras don't fit, the breasts don't stand up anymore, and they have a sunken, hollowed appearance.

Another type of woman who wants her breasts made larger may be younger—she is a woman who just doesn't have a lot of breast tissue. This varies from a woman who is totally flat chested to one who might just feel that her breasts are not in proportion with the rest of her body.

This surgery is particularly personal and sensitive for the patient and the surgeon, because it involves a sexual part of the body. Most women who want larger breasts want to feel more feminine, more sexual—in fact, some women who have this surgery will feel a change in their sexual response, just because they will see themselves as being sexier than before. Such women, who have previously hidden their breasts from their partners, now, with pride in their breasts, feel more sexual. Thus this surgery, in changing the feeling a woman has about herself, is also changing that woman's sexuality.

In augmentation of the breast, the scars are barely visible, a great advantage in breast surgery (in the other two breast procedures the scars are noticeable). A surgeon has the choice of three places to make the incision—in the fold under the breast, in the areola, or in the underarm.

Augmentation of the breast, explains Dr. Glassman, involves the implantation of a bag containing either silicone gel or saline (a salt solution), or both, *behind* the breast tissue or *behind* the muscles of the chest, thereby forcing the normal breast tissue forward. (Contrary to common belief, the implant is not actually in the breast itself.) This surgery does not interfere with the physiology of the breast. Consequently, you can continue to reliably examine your breasts yourself and you can have mammograms.

Although this bag of silicone gel or saline will not move (as silicone liquid can), there is a potential problem in 10 to 30 percent of the women who have this surgery, and that is developing scar tissue internally (which squeezes the breast implant and feels firm to the touch). That is a risk of the surgery but one your doctor may be able to correct.

After the surgery there are some restrictions. Within three or four days, the patient can return to normal, everyday activity because, unlike some other surgeries, the breasts are concealed with clothing. But the doctor will caution you not to drive a car for three to four days; to wear a bra continuously (day and night) for the first week, during the day for the second week, and then whenever you wish (you can even go braless). You must massage your breasts daily in order to keep the body from developing scar tissue. You can't play tennis or engage in other strenuous activity for three to four weeks after the surgery.

• 2. *Breast reduction:* Having very large breasts can cause problems for some women. They may develop back problems later in life (even a curvature of the spine); some develop grooves in their shoulders as a result of the pulling of bra straps; some get rashes under their breasts where perspiration on the skin causes irritation; and large breasts can be painful to carry around. Thus breast reduction for women who wear a DD cup and want to be smaller (it is not recommended for a woman who wants to go from a B cup to an A cup) is a very real option.

But you should be aware that this surgery is a major operation where portions of the breast tissue are used to shape a new breast—the surgeon will remove skin and breast tissue and will relocate the nipple on the new breast. The surgery takes three to four hours to perform; there may be significant blood loss (unlike any other plastic surgery procedure); and the resulting scars are visible. It takes about two weeks to recuperate from this surgery, and you cannot engage in any strenuous exercise for at least a month.

• 3. *Breast lifting:* To lift the breast, the surgeon will remove the excess skin of the breast and relocate the nipple and areola higher on your chest. There is definite visible scarring from this surgery. For many women, this presents a difficult decision—even though their breasts hang down low and they find this unattractive, having upright breasts with visible scars may not be a satisfactory alternative.

STRETCH MARKS (ABDOMINAL LIPECTOMY)

Nothing can really be done to remove stretch marks on the breasts. But for those on the lower abdomen, there is a remedy—what is called an abdominal lipectomy, or a "tummy tuck." Women who have "tummy tuck" surgery are usually thin, have had children, and have stretch marks on the lower half of the abdomen (and some hanging folds of skin in that area). Most doctors will not perform a "tummy tuck" as a dietary measure.

FAT SUCTIONING (LIPOLYSIS)

This operation, pioneered in France, involves suctioning extra fat from under the skin. It is done on the buttocks, the hips, the thighs, the knees, the neck and any other part of the body with extra fat. To be an ideal candidate for this surgery you should be less than thirty-five years old (because your skin still has the elasticity to shrink after the fat has been removed). It is a procedure that should not be done on someone who is fat; it is done on someone who is generally in good condition, whose weight is no problem, but who has fat deposits on some parts of her body. It is major surgery.

Reconstructive Plastic Surgery

Reconstructive plastic surgery is done to aesthetically and functionally correct various problems to return a person to normalcy. Some may be congenital defects—you are born with them—like a cleft palate, a deviated septum or no chin. Also, a prominent, overextending jaw can be reset at a backward slant, not only to improve the appearance but to improve the bite as well.

Other reconstructive surgeries are for people who have had traumas from accidents, many from car accidents. Says Dr. Glassman: "I think some of the worst injuries I have seen have been on women who were not wearing seat belts, who were thrown through the windshield and back—what happens is that the glass breaks on impact and then shears off pieces of the face as the person comes back into the car. Seat belts certainly help."

Another example of reconstructive surgery is neoplastic surgery which is done after the growth of cancers. People who have cancer of the salivary glands, of the jaw and, most commonly, of the skin, may need this type of surgery.

For a woman who has had a mastectomy (done by a general surgeon), the next step, some six months down the road, may be having a plastic surgeon reconstruct a breast. There are several things a plastic surgeon can do. One is to use a breast implant for breast augmentation; another is to use excess abdominal tissue; and the third is to use a muscle from your back—the latissimus dorsi—which is brought around to the front to expand the chest. These are successful operations—a great breakthrough for women who have had cancer.

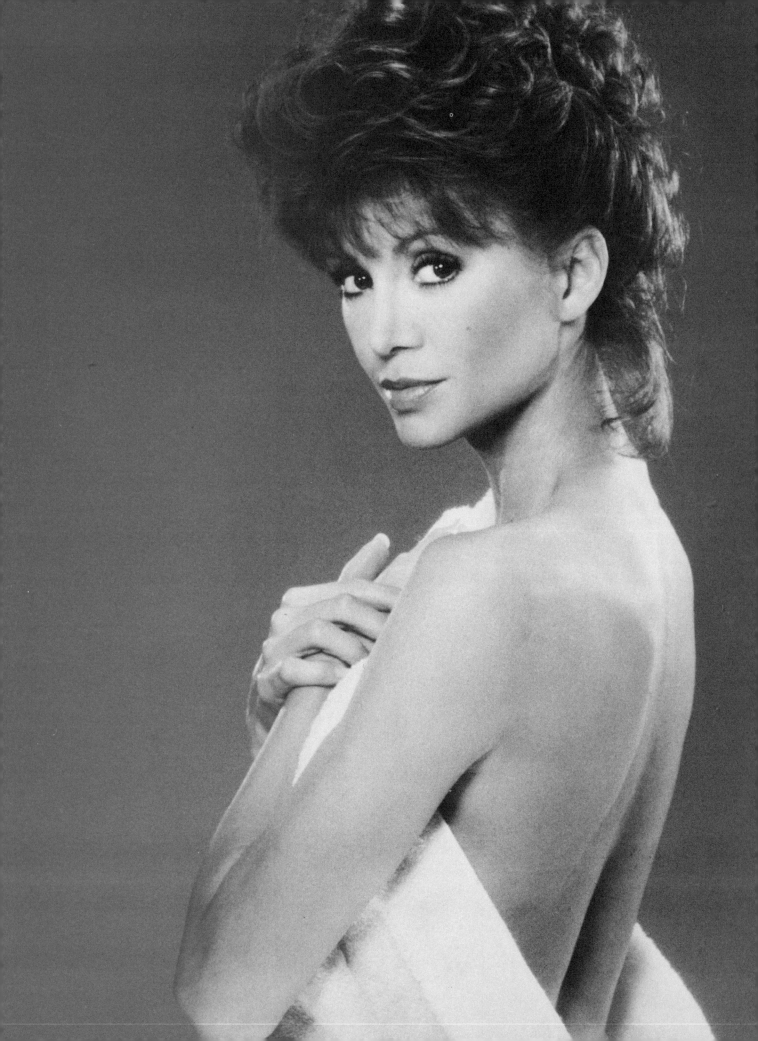

CHAPTER 7

ESSENTIAL LUXURIES

Seems like a contradiction in terms, doesn't it? Something that is a luxury cannot, by definition, be essential, and something that is essential cannot, at the same time, be a luxury. Right? Not always. Although there are priorities in life that are indeed essential for survival—to be fed, to have shelter, to be clothed, to be educated, to work—there are also things that can be considered by some to be luxurious undertakings but that are, at a closer look, actually necessary and important for our bodies to be healthy and beautiful, and for our emotions to be relaxed and content. In other words, essential luxuries are really valuable necessities that significantly affect our inner and outer selves, our total beauty.

I have always believed that, to a certain degree and with perhaps some exception, luxury is in the eyes of the beholder. What may seem like a frivolous undertaking to one person may well be an important part of life for another. But an essential luxury is for everyone. It is getting enough sleep. It is having a massage. It is bathing to relax. It is caring for your teeth, your breasts, your hands. It is something you do for yourself—something to which you are entitled. It is not self-indulgent, narcissistic or selfish. It costs little or nothing—it is simply a setting aside of time to do certain things to care for your

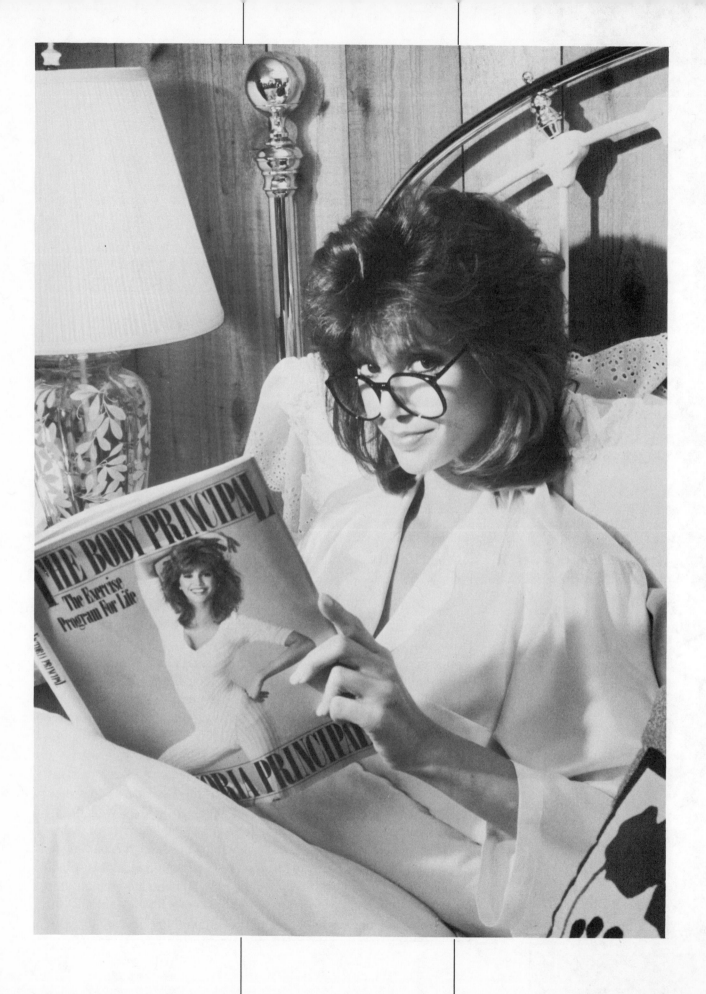

inner and outer needs that will make you a totally healthy and beautiful woman. An essential luxury is simple yet important and becomes a part of your total beauty life affecting all other parts of your life. Whether it's sleeping well (and understanding what a good night's sleep is and how to get it); taking care of your hands, breasts and teeth; getting a massage to soothe aching muscles and a tired soul; exercising to keep your body healthy and toned; or bathing specifically to relax your body and your mind—these essential luxuries result in a totally better you.

SLEEP

It is difficult to feel beautiful, to look beautiful and to act beautiful if you are tired. If you have not had enough sleep, it may be difficult for you to cope with the events of the day. Often on "Dallas" I have a wake-up call for 4 A.M., which means I need to get to bed by 9:30 in order to get a good six hours of sleep; if I don't, I find everything difficult and nothing pleasant. If I don't get what I call "good, solid, uninterrupted sleep," I am edgy, my skin doesn't look and feel fresh, my eyes look and feel "sandy" and stress and fatigue envelop my body. Small tasks take on gigantic proportions; getting through the day becomes irksome and exhausting. Thus, good sleep for me is an essential part of my life. Everyone needs sleep—it is the time when your mind relaxes so it can tackle the next day's challenges. Sleep is essential not only to be able to deal with life but for the body to be healthy and beautiful.

How much sleep do you need? According to Dr. Sonia Ancoli-Israel, assistant director at the Sleep Disorder Center at the Veterans Administration Medical Center in San Diego, California, you need that amount which allows you to function at your highest, most efficient level during the day, and this varies from one person to another. Thus if you are tired during the day, or find yourself not functioning at what you know is your best capability, you may not be getting enough sleep.

People don't get enough sleep for several reasons, but basically there are two kinds of sleep-related problems. One is when you have a hard time falling asleep and/or staying asleep. The other quite common problem is when you find it difficult staying awake during the day usually because you have not gotten enough sleep.

On the other hand, you may feel you are sleeping too much. This is probably due to the fact that you are sleeping inefficiently— that is, your sleep is disturbed, and in the morning you are still tired.

Hints for Getting to Sleep and Sleeping Well

Contrary to what you may have heard, many people can't finish whatever they are doing, fall into bed and immediately fall into a deep sleep. For those of us who, at one time or another, find it difficult to get to sleep, I have found the following suggestions helpful:

1. Go to bed when you are tired. Going to bed early just because you think you need the sleep (and when you are *not* tired) can result in sleeplessness.

2. Make "going to sleep" a pattern, a kind of ritual, where you do the same things every night. Getting into such a routine may help your body "know" that the time for sleep is arriving. For example, about fifteen minutes before I get into bed I turn off all the music and get used to pure silence. I do a short series of stretch exercises. Stretch your body like a cat—relax those tired, taut muscles.

I don't rush. I take off my makeup, and get into a warm shower (or a warm bath). In the shower I do some breathing techniques (slow in's and out's) and a shoulder exercise (hands at your sides, slowly lift your shoulders, now back, then front, up again, then relax). In a bath, I just relax (see Bathing, page 195). Next I do my skin care routine, making sure to moisturize well. (Remember that right before you sleep may be a good time to apply extra moisture and/or medication for your skin.) Then I return to my bedroom, turn down the room temperature (it's more comfortable to sleep in a cool room) and climb into bed. I close my eyes and start relaxing each part of my body starting with my toes and ending with my eyes. That's it.

3. Make sure you sleep on a hard mattress—it is better for your back. If you need a new one and can't afford it, place a three-quarter-inch-thick piece of lumber, the same size as your mattress, underneath it.

4. There is an amino acid in milk (tryptophan) that acts as a natural tranquilizer (or you can take it in tablet form). So try drinking

a glass of soothing warm milk (you can make it low fat for less calories) before you go to bed.

5. If you have a back problem, try sleeping with a bed pillow under your knees. If you prefer sleeping on your side, be sure to keep one knee bent as this takes the pressure off your back. Do not sleep on your stomach—it is bad for your back, and if your face is directly on the pillow, you may be stretching your facial skin.

6. Studies have shown that having sexual relations can make you sleep better.

Dr. Ancoli-Israel recommends the following additional hints for getting to sleep and staying asleep:

1. If you can't sleep, get out of your bed. Your bed should be for sleeping and for loving. If you are tossing and turning, get out of the bed, sit in a chair, read, walk around, but don't get back into bed until you feel sleepy.

2. Get up at the same time every morning. Most people tend to deprive themselves of sleep during the week. It goes this way—you go to bed late, you get up early to take care of the kids or go to work, and therefore deprive yourself of some sleep during the week. When the weekend comes along, you try to make up for this lack of sleep by "sleeping in" in the morning. Then, by the time bedtime comes, you are not tired. So you go to sleep later again, and then the vicious cycle is repeated. Some people can cope with this, but if you have trouble falling asleep at night, then you should avoid this pattern. Force yourself, regardless of what time you go to sleep, to get up at the same time every morning.

3. If you have trouble sleeping at night, avoid naps—they do the same thing: You sleep in the afternoon and you can't get to sleep at night.

4. Avoid caffeine. Studies have shown that it does interfere with falling asleep.

5. Avoid alcohol (this is both for people who have trouble falling asleep and those who have trouble staying asleep). It's an old wives' tale that a glass of wine or sherry will help you sleep. Alcohol will make you sleepy initially, but several hours later, when the alcohol leaves your bloodstream, it wakes you up again. Thus if you

have a drink before you go to sleep, you will fall asleep, but you will wake up at two or three in the morning and will have trouble going back to sleep. Also, if you have a lot to drink after dinner, you may be tired initially but when you are ready to go to bed you will be wide awake. So remember, alcohol causes insomnia.

6. Try reading, or any sort of relaxation exercise. (I do a progressive relaxation exercise—tightening and releasing each part of the body until the whole body is relaxed.)

7. Count your breaths. Breathe deeply, count one breath. Breathe again and count two breaths. After two breaths your mind will wander; bring it back and start counting from one again. Some people who can't fall asleep have active minds that just can't stop going—if that is you, you need to train your mind not to wander. Do this by counting your breaths again. You will soon fall asleep. Progressive relaxation (the previous tip) is good for people who are physically tense. Breath counting is good for people who are mentally tense.

8. Biofeedback has been shown to be great for relaxing. Ask your doctor.

There are some other sleep problems that may be symptoms of a more complex sleep disorder. If you are experiencing excessive snoring, excessive daytime sleepiness (waking up tired, chronic fatigue, falling asleep at inappropriate times during the day) involuntary leg kicking or holding your breath in your sleep, see your doctor. You may have a physiological sleep disorder which can be helped by medical attention.

CARING FOR YOUR HANDS, NAILS AND FEET

Hands

I was born with old hands, and time has continued to age them. But, since I consider hands to be such an important and beautiful part of the body, a part I don't want to hide, I take care of them. Hands are one form of communication (for some of my friends, the *only* form

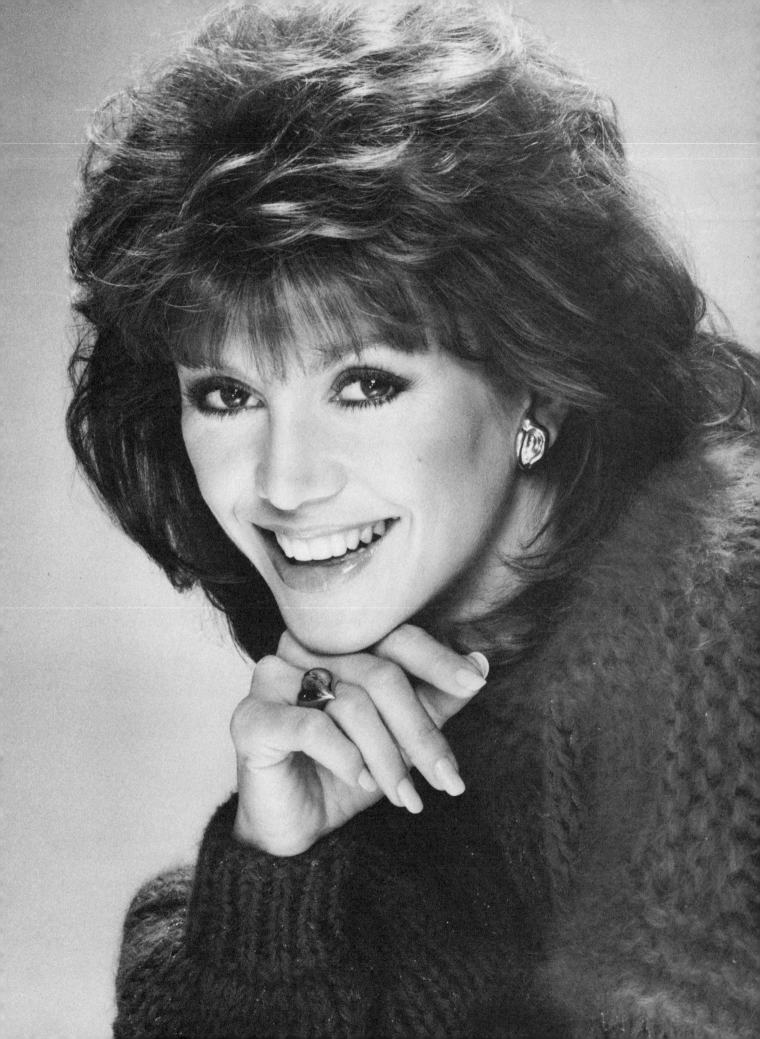

—if you tied their hands behind their backs, they wouldn't be able to speak!). We create images with our hands—gestures that are part of our way of speech. Thus it's a shame when they are uncared for and unattractive. I have often seen a beautiful woman hiding her hands in her pockets or under a napkin at a table, and I know she feels ashamed of how they look. I am always surprised, because caring for them is so simple. It really is easy to make nearly any hands beautiful—but neglect will ruin even the most naturally beautiful ones.

I have always, routinely, taken care of my hands. Such care doesn't take much time, very little money, and the results are, without question, worth it.

Here are some hand care hints:

1. Carry a hand moisturizer in your makeup bag; keep a tube in your kitchen, on your desk (at home and in the office), in the bathroom and in your car. Use it as often as you think of it. I believe that you can't moisturize your hands too much. The wear and tear on your hands is constant because we use them all the time. When you use the cream, massage it four inches above the wrist—your skin can really wrinkle there too.

2. When I shower I use the same soap on my body and on my hands—a gentle, nonabrasive soap. When washing dishes, I *always* wear gloves.

3. When I go out in the sun, I put the same sunscreen or sun block on my hands as I use on my face.

4. Don't put your hands any place you would not put your face. Often we treat our hands with some disdain. We put them into bags full of all kinds of things; we put them into machinery; we reach into oven doors, toy chests, grocery bags, miscellaneous drawers and the like. Be more considerate of your hands. Be careful and be gentle.

5. Lemon juice can make your hands feel and smell wonderful. For some people, lemon is a neutralizer that helps maintain a normal pH balance in the skin. Put it on your elbows too.

Nails

The nice thing about nails is that they grow about one millimeter every week. That means that even if you have been neglecting or abusing them, you now have a chance to reform and pay attention to your nails—and in a month or so, they'll be beautiful. Even though nails are dead protein (sealed with your cuticles), they grow constantly. Crash diets, certain illnesses, anemia and stress can all affect the condition and growth of your nails.

Hands cannot be beautiful without pretty nails—not necessarily long, manicured but at least clean, shaped ones. And the only way to have lovely nails—long or short—is to manicure them at least every other week.

If you find it difficult to grow your own nails, if they chip and break often, there are alternatives. Juliettes (a paper wrapping is placed around the nail), sculptured nails (a wet powder, also used to make false teeth, is molded on your nail and extended to form a new nail covering that has to be filled in as it grows out, about every two to three weeks), silk nails (a silk ribbon keeps the nail strong and pretty) and other techniques are all "false" or "extension" nails that can give you the long nails you always wanted.

To take care of your own nails, you can give yourself a manicure at home, or you can get a professional one. For a home manicure, you will need:

- A small bowl filled with warm water and liquid soap
- Cotton balls
- Polish remover
- Orange stick
- Nail file
- Nail brush
- Cuticle cream
- Nail buff
- Nail polish—color and/or natural base and top coat
- Oil "quick dry"—or vegetable oil from the kitchen

THE STEPS OF A HOME MANICURE
Sit at a desk, sink or makeup table. Put everything you need in front of you so you won't have to reach anywhere in the middle of your manicure.

1. Use polish remover to take off any polish residue on your nails. Dab it on a cotton ball. Replace it with a new one as soon as it has a lot of color on it. There are new nail-polish-removing products you can try. One I like is a jar with a sponge soaked in polish remover—all you do is put your hand in the jar and the nail polish will come off.

2. Clean around and under your nails with your orange stick.

3. Put your hands in the soapy water, and brush with a nail brush. Rinse and then dry your nails with a towel.

4. File your nails even if they are short to get rid of uneven edges and to give them shape. File sideways, and then point the nail file toward the knuckle, and file on top and underneath to get rid of rough edges.

5. Again dip your hands in the soapy water. Rinse and dry.

6. Put cuticle cream on your cuticles, massage, then put your hands back in the soapy water. Leave them there for five minutes. Close your eyes and relax.

7. Take an orange stick and wrap a little cotton on one end. Push back your cuticles—never cut them with a scissor. (If a manicurist ever does that to you—run!).

8. If you have a tear on a nail, you can repair it with nail glue. Put a dot on the nail, let it dry and then file gently with a nail file.

9. You are now ready for polish. Put on one coat of base (colorless polish). Let it dry. Now apply one coat of colored polish, spreading it evenly but not thickly (a little at a time), and let it dry for a few minutes. Be sure to also polish under your nails so they won't be one color on top and another underneath. Now put on another coat of the color, and let it dry. Take the orange stick, dip it in polish remover, and use it to remove the excess polish around the nail. If you don't like colored polish, at least put on two coats of clear polish to protect your nails.

10. Put on a top coat (it is colorless and seals your polish). If you don't have thirty minutes to let it all dry, brush on some "quick dry" or vegetable oil.

11. Periodically during the week you can add as many coats of clear polish as you like. The more, the better—your nails will be better protected.

Feet

Chances are you are like many other women—you don't give your feet as much care as you do your hands, probably because your feet are often covered. But if you think about it, your feet are exposed at home, everywhere in summer months, and always in open-toed shoes. And besides, if you ignore the health of your feet, they'll ache, and you'll feel tired; if they are sore, and you don't massage or otherwise soothe them, your whole body will feel weary and uncomfortable. Feet are as much a part of your body as your hands and they need care.

Once you start caring for your feet—and it is a simple routine—it will become a habit. All you have to do on a daily basis is:

1. Wear comfortable shoes. If you walk a lot, wear walking shoes and leave the four-inch heels for dancing. The rule is—if your feet are comfortable, you will be too.

2. Massage your feet when you take off your shoes—it will soothe your aching muscles.

3. During the day, take off your shoes and flex your feet, then point your toes. Do this ten times, twice a day.

4. When you take a bath, scrub your feet with a loofah, then massage them with a moisturizing body cream.

5. Try giving yourself a pedicure—and you'll be surprised at how lovely your feet will look and how sexy you will feel.

THE PEDICURE

If you've never done it, and if you can afford it (it costs about fifteen dollars), treat yourself once to a professional pedicure at your local beauty salon. You will feel wonderful—and you'll learn the relatively simple techniques you will then be able to do for yourself at home.

For a home pedicure, the equipment you need is the same as for a manicure, plus a bottle of moisturizing body cream and a large bowl or pot of soapy warm water to put your feet in. There are two other options here—one is to use your bathroom sink if it is attached to a counter you can sit on; the other is to buy an electric footbath (available at most drugstores, hardware stores and five-and-dimes) which will keep the water heated (it sometimes also has a built-in foot massage). Here are the steps of a home pedicure:

1. Remove polish from your toenails using cotton and polish remover. Soak your feet in the soapy water for five minutes. This will soften your skin, your cuticles, loosen any dirt in the toenails, and relax your feet. (You can add two tablespoons of lemon juice to the water—it softens the calluses on your feet). If you get bored just sitting there, try some of my exercises for strengthening the ankles (they also stretch the foot muscles). Put your feet flat in the footbath; flex your toes up toward you, then curl them down. Do this ten times. Now pick up your feet entirely (leaving your heels on the base of the bowl), bringing them up and down another ten times. If you have the room, try this ducklike exercise: With your feet ten inches apart, keeping your heels on the base of the bowl, move your toes toward each other, then back. Do this five times. Now take one foot out of the water. Work on this one until you are ready to moisturize; then work on the other.

2. Take a pumice stone and rub your heel and the ball of your foot to remove any buildup of dead skin. In a salon the pedicurist will use a sharp instrument to actually shave callused skin off your feet (she may also do this to your corns). I wouldn't advise trying this at home—it can be dangerous if you don't know how to do it. Scrubbing your feet should suffice.

3. If your nails are long, cut them with a toenail clipper. Otherwise just file them down straight across.

4. Take your cuticle cream and rub it in. Push the cuticles back with your orange stick.

5. Do steps 2 through 5 to the other foot.

6. Take your moisturizing body lotion and give both feet a good massage—rub the balls of your feet, along both sides, and press on the heels. Be sure to rub between the toes. Take your polish remover or alcohol and clean the toes of cream so that the surface of each nail will be ready for polish.

7. Take a piece of tissue and twist it into a rodlike strip. Stick it between two toes, then pull it around the other two toes, then again and again. The tissue between the toes will separate them and help keep them from smudging the polish. You can also buy inexpensive rubber toe separators from your local drugstore or beauty supply house that do the same thing.

8. Take your base nail polish and give your toenails one coat. Now take a color (even when I wear only natural clear polish on my hands, I put a red or pink on my toes). It lends a blush of color to otherwise colorless feet. Put on a second coat, then a top coat (that's the colorless polish).

That's it. Flex your feet—they'll feel surprisingly sexy, and pretty too.

BREASTS

In the past, many women have not paid attention to their breasts unless they were pregnant or had a medical problem. But today, with further education and the realization that breasts need care, more and more women are appreciating the beauty of their breasts and taking the time to care for them.

I believe that caring for our breasts is not only essential (they *need* such care) but may also be lifesaving (you have to be familiar with your breasts, feel comfortable touching them, in order to examine them properly to catch any signs of cancer).

Normally the care that breasts require takes little time. There are general basic things you should remember to do: Wear a bra if your breasts are larger than an A cup; wear a bra *at all times* (and no matter what size you are) when you participate in a strenuous sport; don't go on crash diets where weight gains and losses become routine—that's a sure way to get stretch marks on your breasts and these are permanent; and watch your posture—if it's not good, your breasts will sag more than they have to.

An easy routine can include the following steps:

1. The skin on your breasts is fragile and needs moisturizing often—this is easy to do after each shower or bath, when you are moisturizing the skin on your body. Rub it in gently—the massaging action is good for the muscles in your breasts.

2. There may be hair around the nipples. This is common and normal. If you don't find it attractive, simply pluck the hairs out with a tweezer, always pulling in the direction the hair is growing.

3. You can do some exercises for the breasts. These will not make them larger—but they will strengthen the pectoral muscles (under the breasts) which can make your chest look larger. Try this one: Clasp your hands in front of your chest and hold for a count of three. Push them against each other—you'll feel your arm muscles tighten all the way up your arms and across your chest. Now pull up this position to where your hands are at the level of your forehead and hold for another count of three. Now back in front of your chest, hold, then down in front of your waist, hold, then up in front of your chest again.

Breast Examination

Once a month it is essential—no, crucial—to examine your own breasts for any lumps and to check the nipples for any unusual colored discharge. The best time to do this is three days after your period has ended (during and before menstruation, and during ovulation, the breast tissues and glands are often swollen, making examination at those times uncomfortable and unreliable). Ask your doctor to show you how to examine your breasts; also ask for a booklet from the American Cancer Society illustrating self breast examination.

While checking your breasts, also examine your nipples. If you are not pregnant or breast-feeding, your nipples should not have a discharge—it isn't normal and can be a sign of a hormonal imbalance, infection or sometimes of cancer. If your nipples are discharging a liquid, see your doctor.

One of the most important things I do for my beauty and health is to see a doctor every year. Today's doctors are so sophisticated—their diagnostic techniques, particularly those for breast cancer (mammography, ultrasound, thermography) relieve anxiety and save the lives of many women. You may want to ask your doctor if he or she recommends doing one of these tests on your breasts to have a record of their healthy condition (in case there is ever a question as you get older, you'll have a record for comparison).

TEETH

Caring for your teeth to maintain their health is not an essential luxury—it's an absolute necessity. We all know how important it is to brush at least twice a day, to massage our gums and to use a Water Pik to prevent gum disease, to floss as often as possible, to use mouthwash for bad breath, and to visit a dentist twice a year.

A word about bad breath. Occasional mouth odor is caused by several things, including food lodged between your teeth (that's why dentists urge you to both brush and floss your teeth daily), the build-up of plaque on your teeth and the digestion of certain foods (you've probably noticed that garlic and onions can leave a bad taste in your mouth and often have an offensive odor). For these occasional times of bad breath, brushing your teeth immediately after eating (whenever possible) or using a mouthwash or chlorophyll drops is the answer.

However, if you have more serious bad breath problems, see your dentist to rule out any local dental conditions such as an abcess or an infection. If none of these are found to be the cause, your dentist may then refer you to your doctor to see if your bad breath may be caused by other medical reasons. As for your teeth, let's face it—pretty teeth may seem like a minimally important priority and a vain concern to some. Nevertheless, think for a minute about how you appear to others. When someone sees you, it is your smile they notice, and if you are ashamed of your teeth, chances are you won't smile. Women who are self-conscious about crooked, yellow or stained teeth hide them, and the result is a seemingly unhappy, uncomfortable attitude. So take stock, and if you are unhappy with the way your teeth look, you can start smiling now.

The good news is a million-dollar smile is now available to many women—not only in lowered costs but in new techniques to make your teeth look better. Even if you never had braces as a kid, it is not too late for an adult woman to have cosmetic (or corrective) dental work done on her teeth. According to Dr. Harry Aronowitz, a clinical orthodontist and assistant clinical professor at the University of Southern California School of Dentistry, here are some breakthroughs—ask your dentist which may help you.

INVISIBLE BRACES

If you never had braces as a kid, and need them now (but refuse to walk around with the makings of a car in your mouth), this may be the solution for you. There are now metal braces (called "lingual" braces) that fit on the *backs* of the teeth, and some that are clear plastic and are nearly invisible.

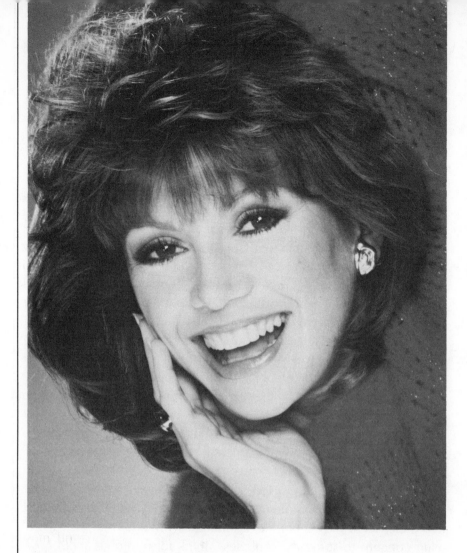

FILING
Filing is so easy, you'll wonder why you never thought of it before! If your teeth are uneven at the edges, your dentist may be able to file them down so tall and short teeth become even.

REMOVABLE ORTHODONTIC APPLIANCES
Dentists now use new variations of what we commonly call "retainers" to help your bite and fix overcrowding of teeth (a retainer holds your teeth in place after the dentist has corrected their position with another appliance). For example, a dental appliance called a "crozat" is often used on adults to move teeth into the correct position. An added plus is that it is removable—you can take it out for dinner parties or photographs. Ask your dentist about the advisability of undertaking dental work to correct problems you may have with your teeth. Remember—you can start such corrective and cosmetic dental work at almost any age.

BONDING
If you broke a tooth as a youngster, chances are you had a cap put on—usually a porcelain cover that fits over a broken tooth and looks just like a real tooth. Now there are other options both for damaged

teeth and for unevenly colored or stained or unequally spaced teeth. In bonding, the dentist paints layer after layer of a liquid acrylic on your teeth (he or she can fill in gaps too), thereby creating a new surface. The process can last up to five years, and can be redone to any individual tooth. But ask your dentist about the drawbacks— teeth can become thicker to the touch, and some can vary in color (particularly if you don't bond each and every tooth).

BLEACHING

This is just what is says—the dentist can remove or lighten some stains on your teeth. It's not a permanent procedure, but it can be repeated.

BATHING

We all know that bathing keeps you clean. What you may forget is that taking a private, calm, warm bath is the cheapest and most beneficial, luxurious relaxation there is. If you take the time to make bathing an experience, you will find it absolutely a must for your well-being, for lowering your stress level, for relaxing completely. It's the most natural of sedatives that can counter the effects of the most harried and exhausting day. Take the time to do it—you deserve it. Here are some hints to help you take advantage of this most wonderful essential luxury:

1. You can instantly turn your bathroom into a Shangri-La. Turn the lights low (you can install a dimmer on your light switch—available in any hardware store—to create a soothing, enveloping atmosphere). If you like candlelight, get six or eight votive candles (you can find them in the supermarket) and place them around the bathtub and/or on your bathroom counter, and turn off all the lights.

2. Put a cleansing masque on your clean (no makeup) face.

3. If you like music, turn on a radio (but don't plug one in and put it on the tub—it's a good way to get electrocuted). Play quiet, soothing, soft music—not blasting disco sounds. Remember, this is the time to wind down, to loosen up, to totally relax.

4. Get into the habit of using a bath pillow. You can buy one at

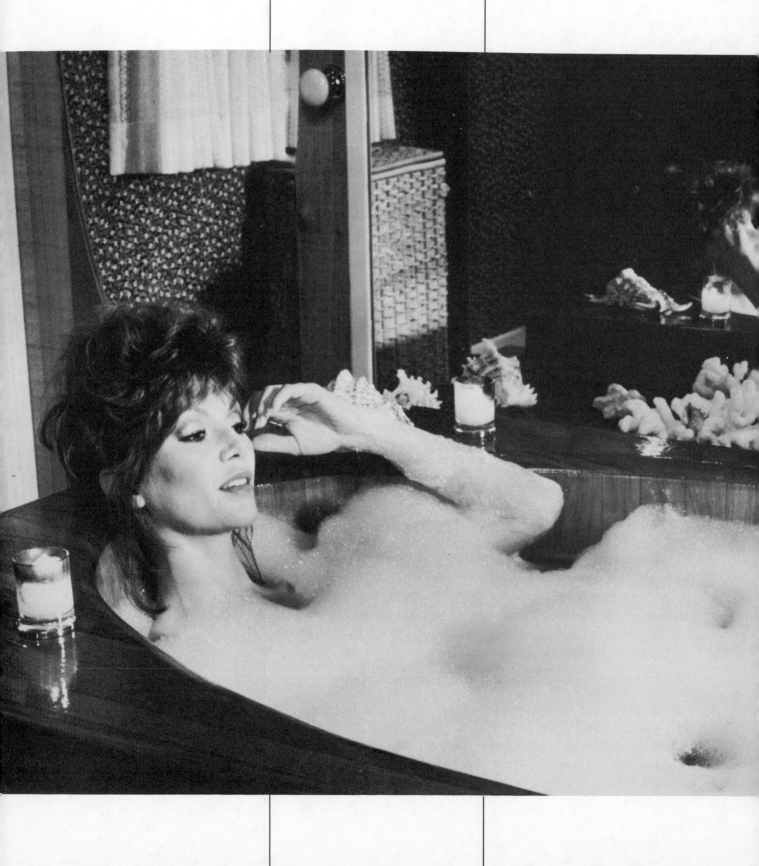

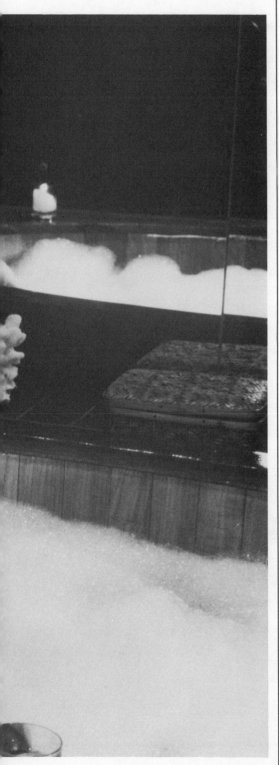

a hardware store (a plastic one usually costs about six dollars). You can also take a soft terrycloth towel, roll it up into a circle (or a rod) and place it under your head. After your bath, you can use it for drying off or to wrap up your hair.

5. Draw a warm bath—not cool, and not too hot (the heat will make your heart race and will drain you of any energy you have left). Don't fill the tub until you are almost ready to get in or the water will be cold. Throughout your bath, as the water cools, add a soft stream of hot water (away from you so you don't get scalded) to keep the water temperature up.

6. Put a few drops of bath oil (or one of those herbal oils found in a health food store) in your tub—it will moisturize your skin. If you like a certain perfume, check if it comes in a bath oil—it's a nice feeling to be surrounded by a fragrance that makes you feel good. You may also want to add herbs to your bath. There are some that stimulate you, others to relieve aching muscles, still others to open up the sinuses.

7. Get into the tub. Close your eyes. Listen to the music. Don't balance your checkbook in your head. Don't go over yesterday's argument with your kids. Don't worry about dinner. Just try an old meditation trick—think of something wonderful and relax. Every so often, test your muscles to be sure they are not tense. After fifteen minutes or so, you can use your washcloth or loofah to scrub off any dead skin on your body (be sure to do the bottoms of your feet and your elbows). I also use a pumice stone on my feet. If you like your back scrubbed, keep a back brush nearby.

8. Keep a plastic cup of mineral water within easy reach. If you feel dehydrated, you can simply reach over and take a sip.

9. Don't hurry out of the tub. But when you feel well rested and rejuvenated, it's probably time to get out. Leave the tub carefully and wrap yourself in a towel or a terry robe. Remove your facial masque with a warm washcloth, then use your astringent and moisturizer (see Chapter 2 for further skin care details).
Obviously, for most of us, taking a relaxing bath may not be possible on a daily basis. But as often as you can, try to set aside a half-hour just for yourself, a private time for thought, for peaceful contemplation, for pleasure, for tranquillity and for relaxation.

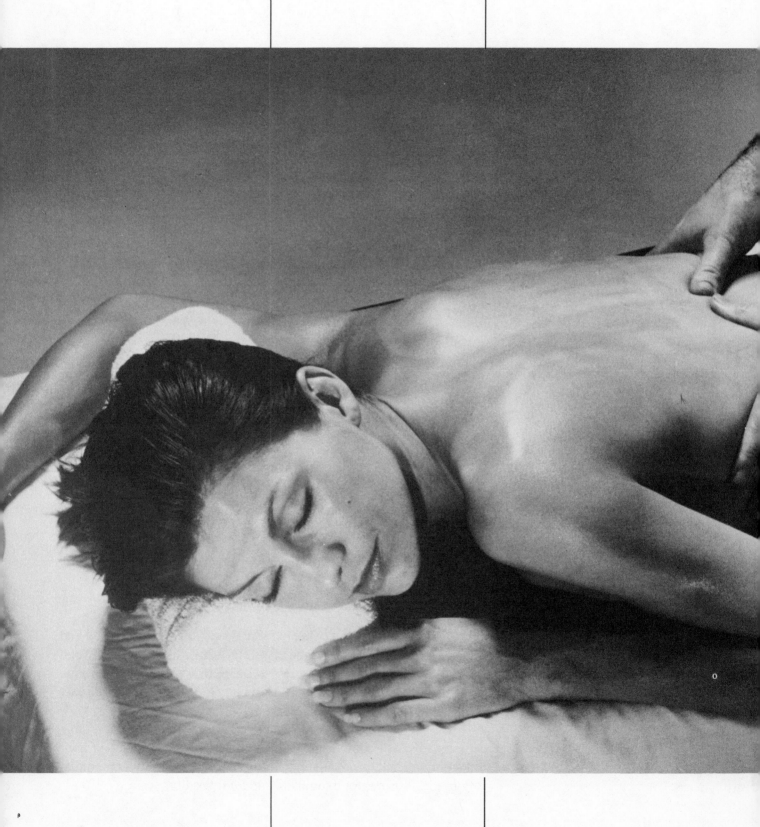

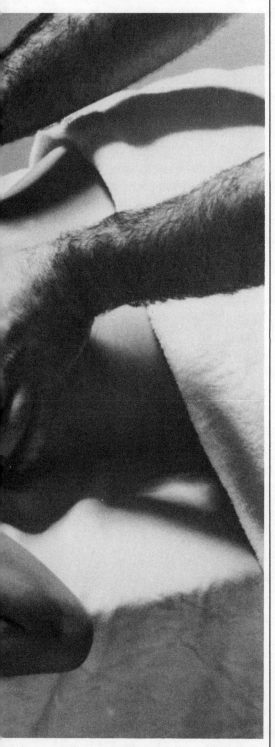

MASSAGE

If you think a long, warm bath is a natural tranquillizer, a totally rejuvenating and invigorating essential luxury, wait until you have a massage. Now there are massages and there are massages. A friend, a husband, a mother can all give you a "massage" of one sort or another. But what I am talking about here is a professional massage given by a licensed masseur, masseuse or therapist who is trained to relieve the pressures and stresses of your day by giving you this experience. A massage is not only a sensual pleasure but is also *good* for you.

If you have never had a massage, it is hard to comprehend its totally relaxing, nearly miraculous soothing powers. It is somehow easier to understand that your muscles will be loosened (extra lactic acid is dispersed, and manipulation and stroking increase the circulation of the blood which, in turn, brings more oxygen to all parts of the body and makes your skin glow).

But I believe it is the emotional and psychological benefits of massage that are so important to our beauty life. In an hour of tranquillity, a masseuse, who is concentrating on making each and every part of you feel better, cares for the health and beauty of your body in a way few others can. On a padded table, in a private room, where the music is soft and the lighting low, a masseuse will take warm oil and, usually starting with your feet, concentrate on working each part of the body so that it is soothed and stimulated in the best possible way. (Of course, a successful massage depends on the skill of the masseuse, so be sure to hire one who is state licensed, if this is required in your state, or who has been recommended by someone you know).

Sounds fabulous, doesn't it? But there are some times when you should avoid massages: if you have just begun to menstruate (your body may be swollen and should not be manipulated), if you have a cold, if you have a skin condition or if you are pregnant. And if you have thin, tender skin that bruises easily, you might want to ask your doctor before embarking on a massage.

For the rest of us, get into the habit. If you can afford it, have a professional massage (it costs between fifteen and fifty dollars for an hour) at least once a year. And, if you'd like, you and your partner can learn the techniques of massage (they are not difficult) so that you can give this essential luxury to each other.

PERFUME

This is an easy essential luxury—easy to apply, easy to store, easily available and easy to use to accentuate and complement your personality. But as easy as it is, some women never got into the habit of using perfume, many forget to put it on, and some just plain overdo it by using too much, everywhere and always. Like many other things, there is method, a reason, a time and a place to use perfume.

What Is Perfume?

Perfume is a fragrance that is either made out of flowers or citrus or spices—and it is these different ingredients that account for the differences in aroma. The term "perfume" means the fragrance in its most concentrated form (it contains alcohol—that's why it is the most expensive). Eau de toilette is less concentrated and less powerful than perfume but stronger than cologne, which is the mildest (and least expensive) form of fragrance. Any may last up to four hours on your body, at which point you may want to reapply it with an atomizer. (I prefer eau de toilette in my atomizer—it is just strong enough for that added touch.)

Choosing a Perfume

I believe there is a fragrance for everyone, and that every woman should select her own basic fragrance; but for many of us, more than one scent gives us a chance to illuminate many sides of our personalities. We may feel mysterious, sensual, innocent, sophisticated, exciting—and can wear a scent to fit each of these moods. But first every woman needs a basic, everyday fragrance that says "This is me," because wearing it makes a statement about yourself. It helps to identify you. Who do you think you are? Are you an earthy, casual, outdoor person—do you like musks, woodsy, spicy or oriental fragrances which are simple, energizing and carefree? Or are

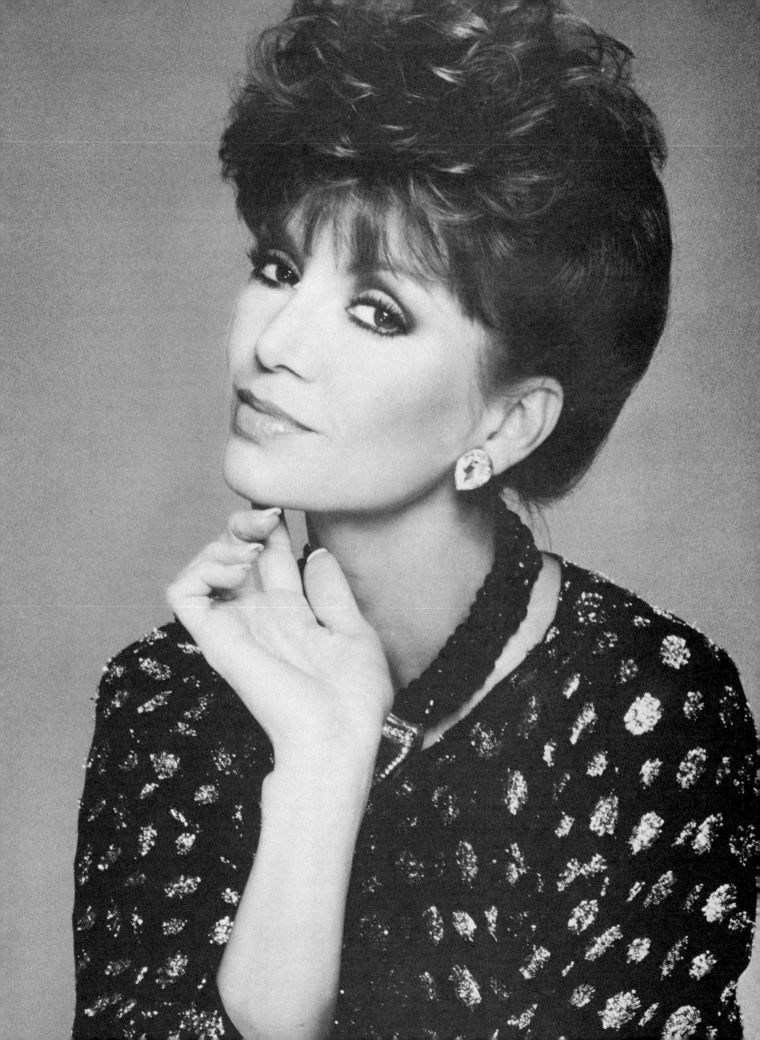

you more like an exotic flower, favoring fresh floral fragrances that are dainty, sweet and relaxing? Or are you a sophisticated woman who wants a clearly identifiable, make-no-mistake-about-it, I-have-arrived fragrance? Your scent can and will represent your self-image.

Fragrance can also affect your mood. I have several perfumes and I wear them at different times depending on how I feel, what I am doing and where I am. When I am in Texas to shoot "Dallas," I wear no perfume because I find that the intense heat changes any scent I wear, and often, after a few hours, makes it offensive. When I do a photo session, I choose a fragrance to match the image I want to present to the camera. My favorite photographer, Harry Langdon, has often greeted me with, "Who are you today?" and then identified me by the perfume he smells. Sometimes after a particular shot I'll change clothes and perfume, and Harry knows that with each new perfume I have a new attitude, that each scent brings out a different part of my personality.

That can happen to you. On the other hand, you can stick to one favorite perfume that you consider to be perfectly representative of who you are. You will quickly become identified with that per-fume—when you leave a room, others will know you were there.

Perfume Pointers

1. Apply perfume sparingly—on your wrists first, then on the sides and base of your neck, on your earlobes or behind your ears, between your breasts. Don't overdo it. You don't want someone to know you are coming before you enter the room.

2. When you apply perfume, never rub it. Let it sit on the skin, so it can be absorbed.

3. Don't just smell perfume out of the bottle. Perfume smells different on every woman—it reacts to the acid and oils in your body to form a scent. So don't expect your best friend's perfume (or the one on the saleswoman in the department store) to smell the same on you. Try it on and walk around for awhile—then smell it again. And always buy a small bottle first (or try the less expensive cologne). If you buy a gallon and then hate it when you get home, you'll be stuck.

4. Perfume is affected by many things. In the summer, heat can

make the scent change—so if you want to keep wearing it, you may want to substitute a lighter version—like cologne. You should know that sunlight can cause the spot where you put the perfume to turn brown, and can make your skin burn more easily.

5. Buy various products—bath oil, powder, body lotion—in the same fragrance as your perfume. You can thus "layer" your fragrance, starting with the soap and bath oil, then the body lotion and/or powder (always powder after lotion), then add the perfume or eau de toilette before you are ready to leave the house.

6. You can add fragrance to parts of your home. Spray it in your underwear drawers or on a tissue or a cotton ball, which you can place in any drawer. When I finish my perfume, I take the empty bottle and put it in my underwear drawer—it keeps its fragrance for some time. I also like fragrant soaps and keep unused bars in my drawers until I'm ready to use them.

7. Never throw away samples of perfumes (unless you absolutely cannot stand the smell). Put them in a purse, one in a stocking drawer and another in your bath water.

8. If you are going to wear a perfume before dinner or before a date, put it on ten or fifteen minutes *before* you're ready, to let it have time to react with your body and to breathe.

9. Even if you love *one* particular scent, have another on hand just for a change.

EXERCISE

This is a whole other book—and I already wrote it. And I quote:

"Where are you going to move when your body wears out? Putting up a 'For Lease, One Body Used' sign is not practical. Neither is trying to make a trade. What happens when our bodies wear out? If we don't exercise, chances are the simplest things in the world will become a strain. It doesn't occur to any of us when we are young that our bodies will not be this strong, this flexible, this shapely forever—not without some help."

The time to take care of your body, no matter how old you are,

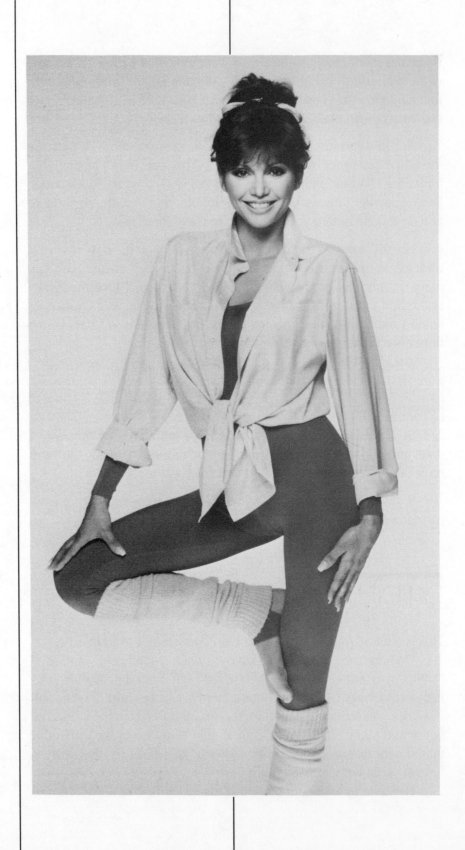

is now. Exercising is essential to survival—and therefore it is not really a luxury. It keeps us healthy and strong. Yet many women are reluctant to undertake an exercise program because they don't have the time, they don't like strenuous classes, they don't want to be intimidated by instructors and exercise fanatics, and they don't know which program is for them. That's why I developed The Body Principal Program—it is the exercise program for everyone, the one program you can do for life. I again quote: "Taking off those flabby thighs or unattractive extra pounds does not have to be difficult or time-consuming. You don't have to submit to daily, hour-long exercise classes, jogging sessions, bike rides, fasting ordeals or sore muscles. Exercise can be easy, affordable, fast, effective and fun. Over the years and out of necessity, I have developed for myself an exercise program that, when practiced in a special, relatively simple way, has become an unobtrusive routine in my life and has resulted in a toned, tight, resculpted body that is in its best condition ever."

Try The Body Principal Program. Or try any other—but exercise. Make it a habit. It is an essential part of your beauty life. All the skin care in the world, all the makeup and hairstyles and massages will be for nought if you neglect your body.

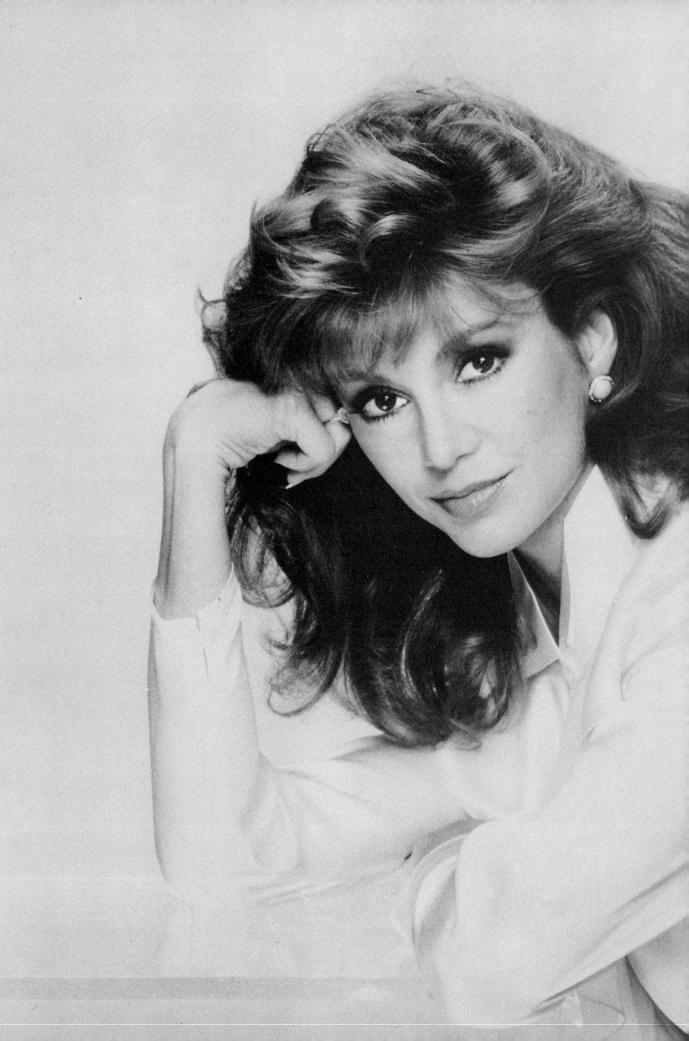

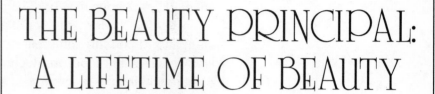

THE BEAUTY PRINCIPAL:
A LIFETIME OF BEAUTY

When all is said and done, beauty is the total you. The totally beautiful woman has made a commitment to taking care of her body, inside and out. She has made room for her own beauty routine in her busy everyday life. She is a woman who understands that, although it is never too late to start taking care of herself, it is better to start young so that a daily beauty program becomes a welcome habit. She believes in her own worth and takes pleasure in her own beauty. She knows that she is entitled to time to care for herself, and appreciates the fact that being beautiful necessitates making a concentrated effort to use this time in a way that is best suited to her life style and needs. She realizes that this means exercising for health and energy, eating intelligent and well-balanced meals, caring for her skin and hair, applying makeup that is becoming and appropriate, wearing clothes with grace and charm to enhance her best features and to radiate an aura of quiet self-confidence. And she is the woman who takes care of herself for herself—she knows that although beauty may be in the eyes of the beholder, it must first exist within herself. This beautiful woman has energy, a sense of self, humor, a generosity of spirit, kindness and is dedicated to making herself the best person she can be. That is a beautiful woman.

Beauty takes work—no one is born beautiful and stays beautiful without it. The Beauty Principal Program makes that time valuable and pleasurable, and the effective results immediately apparent and encouraging. I hope that The Beauty Principal Program for a lifetime of beauty will be for you, as it has been for me, an inspiration and affirmation that with some effort, a little time, a self-awareness, a knowledge of the tools and techniques, and a desire and commitment to making the program a daily part of your life, you too will be the most beautiful woman you can be.

And the next time someone turns to you and says, ''You're beautiful,'' you will know that you really are, inside and out.